AF867327

The IVF Roadmap

Everything You Need to Know Before, During and After IVF in Australia

L. C. Hughes

Contents

Introduction

How to use this book

This book is intended for people who are navigating in-vitro fertilization (IVF) in Australia. Although some of the information may be relevant to those who are overseas, the primary focus is on the Australian system for Australians.

I've organised this book so you can read it start to finish, or skip straight to whatever's in front of you right now.

Part One is the orientation. It covers what to expect, addressing the fears that come up with embarking on this process and how to choose a clinic.

Part Two is about money. I've put this upfront so you can determine if going down the IVF path is even financially possible.

Part Three walks through the actual mechanics of what an IVF cycle looks like and the decisions that need to be made. It also covers special topics such as solo parenting, LGBTQ+ family-building, donor conception, surrogacy and fertility preservation.

Part Four is the human side: the emotional weight, deciding how best to involve the people around you (work, family, friends), and the decision about when enough is enough.

Part Five covers what comes after IVF, whichever way your story goes.

To help you look for a specific term or topic, there's an index at the back, as well as a glossary to help explain some of the jargon used. I've also included key sources for the information contained in this book to assist your further research.

A note on who's talking

I'm a lawyer, not a doctor. Everything in this book that touches biology, medicine, or the clinical process is general education, drawn from Australian clinical sources and government guidance, and checked as carefully as I could manage.

Nothing in this book is a diagnosis or personalised advice, and it can't account for your specific circumstances. Only your own doctor, with your actual results in front of them, can tell you what's right for your body. Nothing here should delay you from seeing one.

The same goes for money: Medicare rebates, Pharmaceutical Benefits Scheme (PBS) thresholds, state schemes, and clinic pricing are described as accurately as I could make them at the time of writing, but these are set and revised by government bodies and individual clinics on a regular basis. Treat every dollar figure in this book as just a starting point for your own conversation with Services Australia, your clinic's billing team, or a financial adviser.

Where this book touches state or federal law it's general information, not legal advice. Several areas such as donor conception and surrogacy are actively under review or reform as I write this. If a specific legal question matters to your situation, please get advice from someone qualified in that specific area.

I've written a lot of this from my own experience: unexplained infertility, a missed miscarriage, countless appointments, invoices and waiting rooms, alongside professional training that made me want to understand the system rather than just survive it. That's the lens this book is written through. It isn't the only valid one, and your own experience may look nothing like mine. I hope it's useful anyway.

Part One

Before You Start

Chapter One

Is It Time?

I found out what a "missed miscarriage" was on a Saturday morning, in a dim ultrasound room, from a sonographer who was very kind and very quiet, which is how you know before anyone says anything.

I was 33 years old and it was the first time that I had ever gotten pregnant. My husband and I had been together over 8 years at that stage, married for 2. We were so ready to welcome a baby into our lives. In the last year we had moved from a one-bedroom city apartment to a house in the suburbs with a backyard. My law career was flourishing: I was just about to be made a partner at a global firm. Everything I had been working towards was falling into place.

Except for this. This, I had no control over. As a high-achieving lawyer I was used to being in control. And I understood almost nothing about what was happening to my own body.

That's really why this book exists. Not because I'm a doctor (I'm not, and I want to be upfront about that from the very start), but because I, like many women, thought that my fertility was just another thing that I could control.

As we embarked on the process of understanding why I was struggling to get pregnant, our tests came back with a so-called diagnosis of unexplained infertility. Unexplained infertility, for us, meant exactly that: every test came back "normal," and there was still no baby. Nobody could tell me why.

In my typical lawyer fashion, I did a copious amount of research online about what I was going through and what I should do next. However, it soon became apparent that the majority of fertility content online, be it forums, social media, or IVF marketing materials, describes a version of IVF that simply isn't how it works today in Australia. IVF is a rapidly changing field globally and a lot of the information out there is outdated, subject to a different regulatory regime or otherwise.

The purpose of this book is to give you, in one place, what I had to piece together myself about the system I was moving through: the money, the process, the choices. Having a basic understanding of that will hopefully provide you with some relief amongst the chaos, confusion and grief.

Embarking on IVF transformed my life. It allowed me to reclaim some of the agency I had lost amidst my unexplained infertility diagnosis. It changed the way I viewed the world: the weight of infertility and fertility treatments caused a dramatic shift in my focus from my career onto my health and my family. And it ultimately resulted in the birth of my much-loved son, and in me becoming a mother for the first time.

Motherhood has been one of the most profound experiences of my life.

There's something I want to be honest about at the outset. I can't tell you what your outcome will be, and neither can anyone else, no matter how confidently they say otherwise.

What I can do is walk you through what I wish someone had walked me through: clearly, without judgement, and without pretending it's simpler than it is.

When to ask for help

If you've picked up this book, you may be in one of two places. Either you've been trying for a while and you're wondering whether "a while" now counts as long enough to do something about it. Or someone (a GP, a family member, your own gut) has already used the word "infertility" near you, and you're not sure what happens next.

Fertility isn't like a broken arm, where the path from symptom to specialist to treatment is obvious. It's slower, murkier, and far more emotionally loaded, which is exactly why so many people either wait too long out of hope, or panic too early out of fear.

The general guidance shared by Australian public health education programs looks like this: if you're under 35 and haven't conceived after 12 months of trying, it's worth starting a conversation with your doctor. If you're 35 or older, that shortens to 6 months, because time matters more to egg quality and quantity from your mid-thirties onwards. If you're 40 or older, most specialists would say don't wait for a timeline at all: start the conversation now.

But please don't treat these as rules you have to earn the right to break. There are situations where the calendar shouldn't matter at all:

- Irregular or absent periods, which can mean ovulation isn't happening predictably, or at all
- A known condition like endometriosis (tissue similar to the uterine lining growing outside the uterus) or Polycystic Ovary Syndrome (PCOS) (a common hormonal condition that can disrupt ovulation), a prior pelvic infection, a previous cancer treatment, or similar
- Two or more miscarriages
- A previous vasectomy, tubal surgery, or similar procedure
- You're not in a situation where pregnancy could happen naturally in the first place: you're single, or in a same-sex relationship, and you know from day one that you'll need assistance.

Before anyone says the word "IVF"

Although IVF is probably the most well known and talked about assisted reproductive technology (ART), it isn't the first rung on the ladder for most people.

Timed intercourse and ovulation tracking is often step one: working out your actual fertile window (which is narrower and easier to miss than most people realise) using tracking apps, ovulation predictor kits, or basic bloodwork, and simply making sure timing isn't the barrier.

Lifestyle review comes up early too. Things like weight, smoking, alcohol, and certain medications affect fertility for both partners, and a good specialist will raise this factually and without shame, because it's one of the few levers you can pull yourself while other things are being investigated.

Ovulation induction, using medication to encourage or regulate ovulation, is a common next step for people with irregular cycles or conditions like PCOS, often combined with timed intercourse, sometimes with monitoring.

IUI (intrauterine insemination) is frequently the step directly before IVF. It involves placing sperm directly into the uterus around the time of ovulation. There's no egg retrieval, no embryo lab, and the process generally involves less medication and monitoring than an IVF cycle. It's typically used for mild male-factor issues, unexplained infertility, single parents or couples using donor sperm, and situations where intercourse isn't part of the picture at all. It doesn't work for everyone, and your specialist will tell you honestly if your situation makes it unlikely to succeed, but it's a real, lower-intensity option with reasonable success rates for the right situation.

Surgical options for conditions like endometriosis, fibroids (non-cancerous growths in or on the uterus), or blocked fallopian tubes sometimes resolve the issue enough that no further assisted treatment is needed at all.

What starting a conversation looks like

Start with your GP, because a GP referral is more useful to you than going directly to a fertility specialist. In Australia, a GP referral to a fertility specialist is valid for 12 months, while a referral from another specialist is only valid for 3 months. Since this affects your Medicare rebate eligibility, getting the longer one from the start saves you time later.

If your treatment is still ongoing past the 12-month mark, you'll need a new referral before it expires. If you know you're likely to be in treatment for well over a year, it's also worth asking your GP directly whether an indefinite referral might be appropriate, given fertility treatment can sometimes qualify as an ongoing condition requiring long-term specialist management.

Your GP can do useful groundwork before you get to a specialist: basic bloodwork, a conversation about your cycle history, and also a semen analysis referral for your partner.

When you get any referral, check it has both your name and your partner's name on it (if applicable). An incorrectly addressed referral is one of the most common, most avoidable reasons rebate claims get delayed.

If you're not doing this the "traditional" way

If you're a single parent by choice, in a same-sex relationship, or building a family through donor conception from the outset, it's worth knowing that this doesn't change your access to care. Medicare rebate eligibility for fertility treatment in Australia is no longer restricted by relationship status, sexual orientation, or gender identity.

Chapter Two

The Big Picture

I've summarised the IVF process from start to finish in eight steps.

Not everyone moves through these steps in a straight line, and not everyone hits all of them. Some people move from testing straight to IVF because their diagnosis makes the earlier steps unlikely to help. Some people's path forks entirely away from IVF at some point: toward donor conception, toward surrogacy, toward stepping back. This roadmap is a general guide, not a fixed itinerary. If yours looks different, that doesn't mean you're doing it wrong.

1. **Deciding it's time.** Usually triggered by a timeline, a known condition, or simply your own readiness. This is a decision point, not a commitment to any particular treatment yet.

2. **Getting referred and choosing who you see.** A GP referral, ideally, gets you to a fertility specialist, allowing you to claim Medicare. You choose a specialist, and by extension, usually, a clinic.

3. **Testing and diagnosis, or the lack of one.** Blood tests, scans, a semen analysis, sometimes more invasive investigations. This tells you and your specialist what, if anything, has been identified, and about a quarter of the time, nothing will be. Either way, this stage informs what comes next.

4. **Treatment options before IVF.** Your specialist will recommend a starting point based on your testing, age, and history. As noted above, timed intercourse and ovulation tracking, ovulation induction, IUI and surgical options may be considered before IVF.

5. **If it's IVF, deciding the approach.** As this book will hopefully make clear, IVF is not a one-size-fits-all approach. If you proceed with IVF, you will need to make decisions

about your treatment approach, including the stimulation protocol, whether to do a fresh or frozen embryo transfer, and whether 'add-ons' such as preimplantation genetic testing (PGT) are appropriate.

6. The IVF cycle. A typical IVF cycle involves a stimulation phase (injecting medication over the course of one to two weeks, with monitoring scans), followed by egg retrieval, fertilisation in the lab, embryo development over several days, the fresh or frozen embryo transfer and then finally, the dreaded two-week wait for a result. Any additional embryos can typically be frozen for future use.

7. If it doesn't work the first time. Statistically speaking most people don't conceive on a single cycle. What follows if a cycle doesn't work is usually a review of what happened, sometimes a change to the protocol, potentially further testing or add-on treatments and either a frozen embryo transfer or a new stimulation cycle.

8. Ongoing decisions. How many cycles to try, when to pause, when to consider a different path: donor conception, surrogacy, or stepping away from treatment altogether. These are deeply personal decisions with no single right answer.

Two things run alongside this whole sequence.

- **Money** (Medicare, the PBS, state government grants, health insurance, out-of-pocket costs); and
- **The emotional weight** (fear, grief, strain on relationships, who to tell and when).

The fears nobody puts on the consent form

There's a form you sign before an IVF cycle starts. It lists risks, procedures, medications, consent for storage and disposal of embryos: everything a clinic is legally required to spell out. I remember sitting with a pen in my hand, reading the clauses like I would have for a client, and thinking: none of this is actually what I'm afraid of.

I wasn't afraid of the clinical risk percentages. I was afraid of the plethora of needles I'd be holding against my own stomach. I was afraid of what it would do to me, to my sense of identity and goals and to my marriage, if this didn't work. I was afraid of my colleagues asking why I kept turning up to work late after monitoring scans and tests. None of that was on the form, because none of it was the clinic's job to cover. It was mine to carry, mostly alone, mostly quietly, for a long time.

I don't think I'm unusual in that. Almost everyone going through this is carrying a version of the same list, and almost nobody says it out loud until it starts leaking out unexpectedly: tears in a car park, snapping at a partner over something unrelated, Googling things at 1am that don't have answers.

Needles. Often the one people are most embarrassed to admit, especially as an adult who feels like they should be past being scared of an injection. You're not being dramatic: daily injections, sometimes more than once a day, for weeks, are a real physical and psychological load.

What the hormones will do to you. Not just physically (bloating, tenderness, fatigue) but the mood volatility that catches so many people off guard.

The procedures themselves. Egg retrieval, in particular, sounds worse in the abstract than most people find it in practice, though "most people" isn't a guarantee for you, and it's fair to want a plain, unflinching account of what actually happens and what recovery looks like.

The two-week wait (or TWW). The gap between transfer and test result carries its own dread: a fear of hoping too much, paired with a fear of not hoping enough to protect yourself. I don't think there's a trick that removes this entirely.

A cycle not working. This is the fear underneath most of the others, if we're honest.

Being found out before you're ready to tell anyone. Sneaking to appointments, inventing reasons for time off, managing your face at a social gathering where someone asks "so when are you two having kids?"

Judgment, real or imagined. From family with opinions about "trying naturally a bit longer," from friends who got pregnant without trying, from your own inner voice on harder days.

What it does to a relationship. The scheduling, the grief that sometimes isn't shared evenly between partners, different coping styles under the same roof.

The money running out before the hope does. This book keeps the money chapters dense and practical because that information matters. But the fear sitting underneath the numbers is real too, and it deserves more than a spreadsheet.

None of these fears mean you're not ready. I had all of them, at one point or another.

As the saying goes: **courage is not the absence of fear, but the triumph over it.**

Chapter Three

Common Myths about IVF in Australia

A huge amount of fertility content online (forums, American media, international clinic marketing) describes a version of IVF that simply isn't how it works in Australia. Some of this is attributable to a variation in medical practice; a lot of it is regulatory. This chapter exists to sort out what actually applies here, because carrying assumptions from an American forum or a UK news story into a conversation with your Australian clinic can lead to some confusing, sometimes disappointing, moments.

"Can I choose the sex of my baby?"

No, not for non-medical reasons, and this is one of the most consistently searched and misunderstood aspects of Australian IVF. Non-medical sex selection (sometimes called "family balancing," choosing an embryo's sex simply because you'd prefer a boy or a girl, unrelated to any medical need) has been banned under national ethical guidelines since 2004. Australian research has found consistently strong public disapproval of non-medical sex selection.

Sex selection is legally permitted here in one specific circumstance: to avoid passing on a serious sex-linked genetic condition to a child, using PGT-M technology, but strictly for medical, not preferential, reasons. If you've read about "family balancing" clinics or seen Australian families travelling overseas specifically for elective sex selection, that reporting is accurate (some families do this), but it's not something available through the Australian system, and no Australian clinic will offer it for non-medical reasons regardless of how the request is framed.

"Does IVF mean I'm likely to have twins?"

This one caught me by surprise. I had always heard about IVF often resulting in twins and multiples. Transferring multiple embryos at once was more common in IVF's earlier decades, partly to improve the odds per attempt, but it also meaningfully increases the risk of a multiple pregnancy, which itself carries higher risk. **Single embryo transfer is now the standard, recommended approach in Australia**, precisely because the evidence shows it produces comparable cumulative success with meaningfully lower risk, when combined with freezing any additional viable embryos for future use. If you've read older or international material describing multiple-embryo transfer as routine, that reflects either outdated practice or a different country's standard of care, not what an Australian specialist will generally recommend as a first approach.

"Can I pay someone to carry my baby?"

No. This surprises many people who've absorbed the American model of commercial surrogacy from film and TV. **Commercial surrogacy is illegal everywhere in Australia**, and altruistic surrogacy (which allows only reasonable expenses, no payment for the pregnancy itself) is the only lawful form nationally. Several states go further and criminalise Australians engaging in commercial surrogacy arrangements even overseas. This is a substantial, deliberate departure from the US model, where commercial surrogacy is legal and well-established in several states, and from a number of other countries that have built entire international surrogacy industries around it.

"Can I pay for eggs or sperm?"

No. Donors can be reimbursed for reasonable, verified expenses, but not paid for the genetic material itself. This is a real point of contrast with the United States in particular, where compensated egg donation is a large, established industry, and donor profiles are often marketed with compensation figures attached. In Australia, the cost of donor gametes typically reflects screening and coordination costs, not a payment for the eggs or sperm themselves, unless they are being imported from overseas.

"Will my donor stay anonymous forever?"

Anonymous donation has been banned in Australia since 2006. Every donor consents in advance to their identity being released to any donor-conceived person once they turn 18. Some other countries still permit or historically permitted lifelong donor anonymity, and donor profiles or sperm bank material sourced from those jurisdictions may be marketed with anonymity as a feature.

"Isn't IVF basically the same everywhere, just with different price tags?"

IVF is not one universal, internationally standardised medical product with only cost varying by country. What actually varies from country to country includes: what's legal, what's regulated and how strictly, the costs involved, and in some cases genuine differences in typical clinical protocol.

Australia consistently ranks among the world's top-tier IVF systems on quality. It is one of the few countries in the world, alongside the US and UK, to track and publish official success rates, whereas most countries lack centralised data to validate performance claims self-reported by clinics.

When evaluating success rates in other countries, be wary of how figures are reported. The Australia and New Zealand Assisted Reproduction Database (ANZARD), managed by the University of New South Wales (UNSW), collects outcome data from every IVF cycle performed across Australia and New Zealand. ANZARD recommends live birth rate per initiated cycle as the most meaningful metric, since it accounts for cancelled cycles and failed embryo transfers. Contrast this to per-transfer rates that can look higher but exclude those failures.

Chapter Four

Choosing a Clinic

This chapter isn't about telling you which clinic to choose. It's about giving you the tools to interrogate the choice properly, the way you'd want to interrogate any major decision involving your body, your time, and a lot of your money.

Before you can make that choice properly, it helps to understand what you're actually choosing between, because "the clinic" and "the doctor" aren't quite the same thing, and the relationship between them is easy to misunderstand from the outside.

In Australia, most fertility specialists are reproductive endocrinologists or gynaecologists with additional training in reproductive medicine, and most operate as private specialists, meaning your actual doctor-patient relationship is with them individually, not with the clinic as an institution. What the clinic (or "ART unit") provides around them is the infrastructure: the embryology laboratory, the nursing team, the reception and admin, the day-surgery facilities for retrievals, and the RTAC accreditation that governs how the whole unit operates.

This matters for a few practical reasons:

- **A specialist may practise at more than one clinic or location**, sometimes within the same group, sometimes even across different ownership groups. If you choose a doctor first, confirm exactly which location(s) they consult and operate from, since that affects your travel and scheduling.

- **The lab and clinical team stay largely constant even if your doctor doesn't.** If your specialist is away, unwell, or on leave during a critical moment in your cycle (retrievals and transfers are time-sensitive and can't simply wait), you'll usually be seen by a covering doctor from the same clinic. If a fair question to ask who will cover for them in those circumstances.

- **You'll interact with more people than just your specialist.** A fertility nurse coordinator is often your actual day-to-day point of contact: booking scans, answering medication questions, talking you through injections. Embryologists run the lab work and will sometimes speak with you directly about your embryos' development, particularly around transfer decisions. Sonographers perform your monitoring scans, which may or may not be with your specialist directly. A fertility counsellor is typically available as part of standard care, sometimes required at certain points (for instance, before using donor gametes). Understanding this team structure upfront means you're not caught off guard when the person calling you isn't the doctor whose name is on the door.

Getting a GP referral

Your GP will usually suggest a specialist, sometimes because of an existing relationship, sometimes because it's the nearest clinic. Neither of those is a bad reason, but neither of them is a *sufficient* one either; you're entitled to do your own research on the doctor, not just accept the referral as final.

It's completely normal to ask your GP for more than one option. This is a relationship you may be in for a while, so it's important to pick someone you trust.

Also, you're not obligated to stay with the first specialist you see if the fit isn't right; plenty of people switch clinics partway through their journey, and a good clinic won't take it personally.

Several major fertility clinics also run their own in-house fertility GP services: a GP who works specifically within, or closely alongside, the fertility clinic itself. The initial consultation is often bulk-billed and they will then refer you internally to one of the clinic's specialists. It's often a faster on-ramp to the process compared with waiting for a routine GP appointment elsewhere.

Where to check success rates

If you remember one website from this chapter, make it **YourIVFSuccess.com.au**. It's run by the National Perinatal Epidemiology and Statistics Unit at UNSW, funded by the Australian Government, and it's the only independent, centralised source of IVF clinic success rates in the country. Every RTAC-accredited clinic's data is calculated the same way, using the same national dataset, rather than each clinic marketing its own preferred numbers. It also has a Patient Estimator tool that gives you a personalised chance-of-success estimate based on your own age and history.

How to read a success rate

"Success rate" can mean at least four different things, and they are not interchangeable:

- **Success per embryo transfer**: the rate people are shown most often, and the most flattering number for a clinic, because it excludes every cycle that didn't make it to transfer at all.
- **Success per started cycle**: a more honest baseline, because it includes cycles that were cancelled or didn't produce a viable embryo.
- **Success per patient, cumulative across multiple cycles**: arguably the most useful number for you personally, because most people don't get pregnant on their first attempt, and this reflects the real-world experience of trying more than once.
- **Live birth rate vs. clinical pregnancy rate**: a clinical pregnancy (a positive scan) is not the same as a live birth, and a small but real gap exists between the two.

It's worth noting that a clinic's overall success rate reflects the patients it treats, not just the skill of its team. A clinic that takes on a higher proportion of complex, older, or previously unsuccessful patients from elsewhere will show a lower headline number than a clinic that mostly treats younger patients on a first cycle, and that doesn't necessarily mean the first clinic is worse. In fact, if you are in a higher complexity category, the first clinic may be more aligned with your needs.

What I would recommend is this: use YourIVFSuccess to get an apples-to-apples national comparison and your own personalised estimate on your Patient Estimator tool, and then bring both to your first consultation and ask your specialist to walk you through what it means for your specific situation.

Choosing a specialist

Another way of going about the process of picking a clinic is to pick the specialist first based on online reviews. This is often more emotionally honest than starting from a spreadsheet of clinic success rates, because a review from someone who's been through it tells you something a clinical statistic can't: how a doctor actually communicates, how rushed appointments felt, whether questions were welcomed. The caveat to this is that reviews are shaped by individual experience and outcomes in ways that can be hard to separate from the doctor's actual clinical skill (someone whose cycle worked is more likely to leave a glowing review regardless of how it was handled, and vice versa). Use reviews to build a shortlist and get a feel for communication style, and then test the fit for yourself at your first consultation.

The clinic cost tiers

This is where clinic choice and money stop being separate conversations, so let's have it properly now rather than waiting to deal with this in Part Two.

Broadly, you're choosing between three tiers, and the difference isn't just price: it's a trade-off between cost, specialist continuity, and time, and it helps to understand all three before you assume the cheapest or most expensive option is automatically right for you.

Standard private clinics are the majority of the market: Genea, Monash IVF Group, the Virtus Health network (which includes IVFAustralia, Melbourne IVF, Sydney IVF, and TasIVF), City Fertility (owned by CHA Medical Group), Queensland Fertility Group, Flinders Fertility, and various independent and regional providers. A standard cycle fee at these clinics typically sits somewhere in the $6,000 to $9,500 range before Medicare, with out-of-pocket costs after rebates usually landing between approximately $4,000 to $8,000 per cycle, depending on the clinic and your specific treatment. Private doesn't mean there are no Medicare rebates: it just means the clinic sets its own fees above what Medicare provides. What you're generally paying for at this tier is continuity with a specific chosen specialist, more consultation time and flexibility, and typically the shortest wait from decision to first cycle, often just weeks.

Lower-cost, bulk-billed private clinics are actually a distinct model, not just a discount on the standard tier. They typically offer a simplified, more standardised treatment protocol, often a rotating pool of doctors rather than one consistent specialist, and tighter appointment scheduling. The clinical process itself (the lab, the embryology, the accreditation) meets the same national standard regardless of tier.

One caveat worth flagging before the clinic-by-clinic detail: "bulk-billed IVF" gets used loosely across the industry. Some clinics bulk-bill particular consultations or services while still charging a gap for the cycle itself; others offer a fixed, low-gap fee for the whole cycle. Whichever clinic you're comparing, always check exactly what's included. Things like medications, the anaesthetist, embryo storage, genetic testing, and other add-ons are very often billed separately on top of the headline number.

Adora Fertility was the first Australian provider to offer bulk-billed IVF, and now runs clinics in NSW, VIC, WA, and QLD. Typical out-of-pocket cost per cycle sits around **$2,500**, against an average of approximately **$8,200** at full-fee clinics. First appointment wait times run around 2-3 weeks, which is comparable to a standard private clinic wait.

There are now numerous bulk-billed, low-cost options run by private clinics such as The Fertility Centre, First Step Fertility, Life Fertility Clinic, and Connect IVF, with prices generally ranging from around **$1,000 to $3,000** per cycle.

Things to know before choosing a low-cost clinic

Here's something to keep in mind before you get your hopes up on a headline price: the low-cost, bulk-billed model generally isn't open to everyone unconditionally. It works financially because the clinic can run a simplified, standardised protocol: fewer drug variations, less individually tailored dosing, and in some cases in-clinic sedation instead of a day-hospital general anaesthetic.

In practice, this usually shows up as BMI and age eligibility criteria for the standard low-cost pathway, alongside general clinical suitability. The criteria are set at a clinic and case level, based on what a simplified protocol can safely and effectively support, and they're not identical across providers or locations.

What this means practically is that you should not assume the lowest advertised price applies to you before asking directly. Ask the clinic what their current criteria are for the standard low-cost service, and what the next-tier option looks like if you don't fit. Getting a clear answer early avoids the frustration of budgeting around a headline number that was never actually available to you.

Lower-cost clinics can be an excellent option, particularly if you:

- are younger with a straightforward diagnosis;

- mainly need standard IVF/ICSI;
- are likely to need multiple egg collections and want to reduce financial pressure; or
- do not require complex genetic testing or highly individualised protocols.

However, ask specifically about:

- the availability of add-ons such as PGT-A (discussed further in Chapter Seven) - many low-cost clinics do not include this, and some may not offer it routinely;
- whether you have access to the same fertility specialist throughout treatment; and
- how stimulation protocols are individualised.

Publicly supported government IVF programs

If you're based in New South Wales, a handful of clinics are publicly supported under the NSW Affordable IVF Initiative, where eligible patients have out-of-pocket costs capped at $1,000 for an IVF cycle after Medicare. These include the Westmead Fertility Centre, Royal Prince Alfred Hospital IVF Clinic, and the Fertility and Research Centre at the Royal Hospital for Women. The level of service, including time and specialist continuity, varies depending on the hospital.

At the time of writing, Victoria is the only state that provides completely free public hospital IVF. However, there are meaningfully longer wait times: often many months from referral to first treatment, since public capacity is limited and demand is high. Continuity with a single doctor is typically lower here too.

Victoria's public fertility care program also sets its own specific age criteria:

- Access to start IVF using your own eggs generally closes at **46 years of age**
- Embryo transfers using previously frozen eggs, embryos, or donor eggs are generally permitted up to your **51st birthday**
- If donor eggs are being used, the donor's egg must be **42 years or younger** at the time of collection

In summary, the estimated cost of a cycle depending on whether you go private, low-cost or a publicly supported route are as follows:

Type of clinic	Estimated cost per cycle (before add-ons)
Standard private	~$4,400-8,800
Low-cost / bulk-billed private	~$1,000-3,000
Publicly supported (NSW govt-backed clinics)	$1,000 (capped)
Public hospital program (VIC only)	$0 (free)

Questions to ask at a first consultation

A few questions that are worth asking a clinic, beyond the obvious ones about cost and timelines, are:

- "What would my personalised, rather than clinic-average, chance of success look like, based on my age and history?"
- "How many cycles do most patients like me need before a live birth, not just a positive test?"
- "What happens if this protocol doesn't work? Is there a defined next step, or do we reassess from scratch?"
- "Who do I actually speak to between appointments if something changes or I have a question? Is there a nurse coordinator?"
- "Based on my situation specifically, would you recommend add-ons such as PGT-A, and why, and is it done at your clinic?"
- "What does your team do to support the emotional side of this, not just the

clinical side?"

It should be remembered that the cheapest IVF cycle is not necessarily the cheapest path to a baby. The goal is not to minimise the cost of one cycle, but to minimise the total cost of achieving your family goal. A low-cost clinic may be ideal for a straightforward case, while someone needing PGT, donor treatment, recurrent miscarriage investigations, or complex male-factor treatment may benefit from a clinic with broader services.

The clinical credentials matter and so do the numbers, but the relationship with your specialist matters just as much. You may be seeing this person, or their team, regularly for months, sometimes years, through some of the hardest news you'll receive. Pick someone you can be honest with and who answers your questions without making you feel like a nuisance for asking them.

A note on the provider list: clinic ownership, pricing tiers, and program names change as the sector consolidates. This list is a starting point for your own research, not a current, exhaustive, or endorsed directory.

Chapter Five

Understanding Your Diagnosis (Or the Absence of One)

Infertility isn't a single condition with a single cause. It's a catch-all term for a wide range of underlying issues: some structural, some hormonal, some genetic, and some that never get identified at all despite thorough testing.

The causes split roughly evenly between the two partners in a relationship: about a third of cases involve a female-factor cause, a third involve a male-factor cause, and the rest are either a combination of both or remain unexplained. This chapter walks through what those causes may look like, and the tests involved to find them out.

Female factors

Ovulation disorders: most commonly caused by polycystic ovary syndrome (PCOS), where irregular or absent ovulation means an egg isn't reliably released each cycle.

Blocked or damaged fallopian tubes: often the result of a past pelvic infection, surgery, or endometriosis, preventing sperm and egg from ever meeting.

Uterine or structural issues: fibroids, polyps, or scar tissue inside the uterus, which can interfere with implantation even when fertilisation happens normally.

Endometriosis: tissue similar to the uterine lining growing outside the uterus, both a structural and inflammatory cause.

Adenomyosis: a condition related to endometriosis, where similar tissue grows into the muscular wall of the uterus itself, rather than outside it.

Diminished ovarian reserve: a natural decline in egg quantity and quality that accelerates with age.

Hormonal imbalances beyond ovulation: particularly thyroid dysfunction and elevated prolactin, usually picked up in standard hormone bloods.

Male factors

Blocked or absent vas deferens: the tube that carries sperm from the testicles, either blocked or missing entirely.

Low sperm number or poor sperm production: fewer sperm than expected, or sperm that aren't being produced consistently.

Abnormally shaped sperm: a high proportion of sperm with irregular morphology.

Failure of sperm production: a more complete absence of sperm production altogether.

Anti-sperm antibodies: where the immune system mistakenly targets sperm.

Sperm DNA fragmentation: damage to the genetic material inside sperm .

In rarer cases, an underlying genetic condition, such as cystic fibrosis, or a chromosomal abnormality, is behind it, and some men have a more specific hormonal cause, such as low testosterone or another reproductive hormone imbalance.

How this gets diagnosed

Testing looks different depending on which of the causes above your specialist is checking for.

For women:

AMH (Anti-Müllerian Hormone): a blood test estimating egg quantity.

Other hormone bloods: FSH, LH, TSH, prolactin, and sometimes oestradiol, usually taken early in your cycle.

A pelvic ultrasound: checks the ovaries and uterus, including antral follicle count, another marker of ovarian reserve.

A hysterosalpingogram (HSG), or sometimes a saline sonohysterogram: an X-ray or ultrasound-based procedure checking whether your fallopian tubes are open and your uterine cavity is a normal shape. More invasive than a blood test or standard scan.

Hysteroscopy or laparoscopy, if indicated: surgical, done under anaesthesia, usually only ordered if something specific needs a closer look. Not part of a standard first round of testing for everyone.

For men:

Semen analysis: the central test, looking at count, motility (how well the sperm move), and morphology (their shape). Usually the starting point before anything else is ordered.

Hormone bloods: testosterone, FSH, and LH, checking whether a hormonal imbalance is affecting sperm production.

Scrotal ultrasound: checks for structural issues such as a varicocele (enlarged veins in the scrotum), blockages, or other physical causes affecting sperm production or transport.

Sperm DNA fragmentation testing: not routine, but may be suggested for recurrent miscarriage, unexplained infertility, or repeated unsuccessful cycles, since a standard semen analysis doesn't detect DNA damage inside otherwise normal-looking sperm.

Surgical sperm retrieval (TESE/PESA), if needed: for azoospermia (no sperm in the ejaculate), a specialist may recommend retrieving sperm directly from the testicle or epididymis, both to confirm whether sperm are being produced at all, and to collect sperm for use in IVF with ICSI if they are.

For both:

Genetic screening may also come up for either partner, particularly with a family history of an inheritable condition or recurrent miscarriage.

What the results can and can't tell you

I want to flag something that took me a while to understand: these tests are good at telling you *that* something might be a factor, and not always good at telling you *why*, or what to do about it with certainty. AMH estimates quantity, not quality. A "normal" HSG tells you your tubes are open, not that fertilisation and implantation will happen smoothly. A semen analysis can show clearly reduced counts or motility, and still not explain everything about why conception hasn't happened yet.

This is part of why the process can feel maddening if you're used to problems having clean, discoverable causes. Fertility testing narrows things down. It doesn't always solve them.

When nothing shows up

Approximately a quarter of cases end up being labelled as **unexplained infertility**: every test in the standard workup comes back within normal range, and pregnancy still isn't happening.

Ours was one of them.

Here's what I'd want you to know if you land here too: it doesn't mean the testing was pointless, and it doesn't mean nothing is wrong. It means current testing can't identify what, which is a limitation of the tools. It's also not a dead end, as treatment can, and does, proceed without a named diagnosis. If you and your specialist agree that assistance makes sense, based on your timeline, your age, your history, or simply your own informed choice, that's grounds to move forward. You don't need to earn your way into treatment with a "real" answer.

Why age actually matters

Age comes up constantly in this process. The biological reason age matters for women comes down to eggs, not embryos or the uterus. Every woman is born with all the eggs she will ever have, and that finite pool declines in both number and quality from birth onward, with the decline accelerating sharply from the mid-30s. Unlike sperm, which the body produces fresh on an ongoing basis, eggs have been sitting in your ovaries since you were born, and the machinery responsible for dividing chromosomes correctly becomes progressively less reliable the longer an egg has been waiting. The practical result is a rising rate of chromosomal abnormality (aneuploidy) in older eggs, which is the single biggest reason IVF success rates fall with age, and why so many pregnancies in older women end in early miscarriage rather than failing to conceive at all.

There are some stark statistics in this regard. Live birth rates per IVF cycle using a patient's own eggs are commonly cited at somewhere around 20-26% for women aged 30-34, dropping to somewhere between 1% and 2.4% per cycle for women over 44.

Donor eggs meaningfully reset this calculation. For a woman over 40 using an egg from a donor under 35, success rates for that specific cycle tend to track closer to what would be expected for the donor's age group, not the recipient's.

This is an important piece of context if age-related decline in your own eggs is the primary factor at play in your situation.

Many private clinics set their own upper age limits for treatment using a patient's own eggs. This is commonly somewhere in the vicinity of 46, though some clinics explicitly market having no age cutoff at all as part of their approach. A clinic might allow continued embryo transfers using already-frozen eggs or embryos, or treatment using donor eggs, up to a later age (sometimes around 52) even after closing off new treatment cycles using a patient's own eggs at a younger cutoff.

If the odds of having a successful birth for your specific age bracket aren't what you hoped, there are still real paths forward:

- **Donor eggs** is the most direct lever. As noted above, success rates track the donor's age rather than yours, effectively resetting the calculation.

- **Banking embryos across multiple cycles** allow people to do several cycles to build up a pool of embryos before too much time passes, before attempting a transfer.

- **PGT-A testing** won't create more good eggs, but can reduce the number of miscarriages and failed transfers on the way to finding an embryo that works.

None of these make the odds simple, but they mean "the numbers aren't in your favour" is a starting point for a conversation with your specialist, not a closed door.

What comes next

Whatever your results show (a clear factor, a partial picture, or nothing at all), the next real decision point is usually about treatment options, not more testing. As flagged earlier, you may be offered other solutions before proceeding down the IVF path, such as ovulation induction or IUI.

Ovulation induction

This is medication to trigger or regulate ovulation, for people who aren't ovulating regularly, most commonly those with PCOS. However, ovulation induction is also used to improve the odds when the cause is unclear.

Letrozole and **clomiphene citrate** are the usual starting tablets, both prompting the ovary to develop and release a mature egg. Letrozole is now the preferred first choice for PCOS specifically, since pregnancy rates tend to be somewhat better than with clomiphene. If tablets alone don't work, or a stronger response is needed, **gonadotropins** (injectable FSH-based medication, the same category used in full IVF stimulation) are the step up. They're more effective but need closer monitoring, since they carry a higher chance of releasing more than one egg at once.

Whichever medication is used, your cycle is tracked with ultrasound scans (which are used to track follicle growth) and sometimes urine LH testing, so your specialist can recommend the timing of intercourse, insemination, or a trigger injection (a shot of hCG that completes egg maturation about a day later).

IUI (Intrauterine Insemination)

Prepared sperm is placed directly into the uterus around the time of ovulation, shortening the distance sperm has to travel, without the egg retrieval, lab fertilisation, or embryo culture of full IVF.

Who it suits: mild male-factor issues (lower sperm count or motility, not severe enough to need ICSI), unexplained infertility, donor sperm situations (solo parents, same-sex couples, or couples needing donor sperm for medical reasons), and sometimes mild endometriosis where the tubes are still open. It's generally not used where tubes are blocked, since it still relies on fertilisation happening naturally inside the tube; IVF is the more appropriate step there.

How it works: IUI can run on a natural cycle (no medication, if you're already ovulating predictably) or alongside ovulation induction, monitored the same way as above. Once a follicle is mature, a lab technician prepares the sperm sample ("washing" it to concentrate the healthiest, most motile sperm) and a clinician passes a thin catheter through the cervix to place it directly into the uterus. The procedure takes a few minutes, feels similar to a pap smear, and most people are back to normal activity the same day.

Cost: typically cheaper than IVF, since it uses far less medication and no lab work. Typical out-of-pocket cost after the Medicare rebate is **$3,500-4,000** for a medicated cycle at a standard private clinic, varying by how much monitoring and medication your specific cycle needs.

How many cycles before moving to IVF: there's no universal number, but three or four well-timed IUI cycles is a common benchmark before deciding whether to move to IVF, if pregnancy hasn't happened. Your specialist may suggest fewer if your diagnosis makes IUI a lower-probability option from the start, or more if things are going smoothly with no clear reason to change course. It's a collaborative call between you and your specialist, informed by age, diagnosis, and how you're both feeling about the timeline.

When a specialist suggests IVF from the outset

If IVF is recommended over IUI or ovulation induction straight away, common reasons include more severe male-factor infertility, blocked or damaged tubes, lower ovarian reserve where time matters more, or age-related factors where a specialist judges the earlier steps aren't a good use of your time.

Some of these scenarios also come with a specific IVF add-on already flagged at this early stage.

Severe male-factor infertility may point toward using ICSI rather than conventional insemination from the first cycle. Lower ovarian reserve or age-related factors are sometimes accompanied by a conversation about PGT-A, since the odds of a chromosomally normal embryo become more relevant sooner.

Part Two

The Money

Chapter Six

Medicare and the Real Cost of IVF in Australia

When organising this book, I decided to put the issue of money near the start, rather than later on.

When you're in the middle of an almost-existential crisis like infertility, money is typically the last thing on your mind. I was willing to throw everything, including the kitchen sink, at the problem. I just wanted a baby.

I've seen stories about people who've spent hundreds of thousands of dollars and have no baby to show for it. It's truly heartbreaking: not only do they have to live with the pain of infertility, but also with the ongoing financial consequences, sometimes significant debt that lasts years.

That's exactly why I think money deserves to be covered up-front. A baby is life-changing, but the amount you could end up investing to get there can be life-changing too, in the worst possible way. It can affect every other part of your life.

Knowing your financial limit from the outset is genuinely hard. The desire for a baby can be so strong that nothing else feels like it matters. I don't think there's a formula that resolves this. But working out where your limit sits in a calm moment, together with your partner if you have one, is a very different experience from making that same decision after an unsuccessful cycle, under financial pressure, with your emotions still raw. We come back to this decision (when to pause, when to stop, when to change direction entirely) properly in Chapter Twenty-Three.

The headline number

A standard IVF cycle in Australia typically costs somewhere between **$8,000 and $15,000 before any rebates**, with out-of-pocket costs after Medicare usually landing between approximately **$4,400 and $8,800**, averaging around **$6,900** across a broad sample of RTAC-accredited clinics. Most people need more than one cycle, so a realistic total budget for two to three attempts sits somewhere in the **$15,000-$25,000** range, though your actual number depends on your specific treatment, your state, and whether you are going through a low-cost clinic.

How the Medicare rebates works

"Medicare covers it" doesn't mean you'll pay nothing. Medicare pays back part of a set price determined by the government, called the **schedule fee**, for a given item. Not part of whatever your clinic actually charges. The gap between what your clinic charges and what Medicare covers is yours to fund, unless a safety net or a state scheme steps in.

Specialists are allowed to charge more than the schedule fee, and in fertility medicine, they usually do: schedule fees often sit well below what a procedure really costs to deliver.

Bulk billing may be available for GP visits, but beyond that expect to pay out-of-pocket even where the clinic markets itself as bulk-billed.

An IVF cycle is comprised of separately defined items on the Medicare Benefits Schedule (MBS), each with its own schedule fee and rebate. The actual items are worth knowing, because they explain a few things that otherwise look like inconsistencies on your invoice.

Before the cycle starts, your specialist consultations and any diagnostic testing (bloods, an initial pelvic ultrasound, a semen analysis) are billed under ordinary MBS consultation, pathology, and imaging items, each with the standard rebate (generally 85% of the schedule fee for services provided outside a hospital). These are separate from, and in addition to, the IVF-specific items below.

Once a stimulated cycle begins, most of it is billed under a number of IVF-specific MBS items:

What it covers	MBS item	Schedule fee	Medicare benefit
First cycle in a calendar year	13200	$3,628.90	85% = $3,524.40 (out-of-hospital rate)
Second or later cycle in the same calendar year	13201	$3,394.45	85% = $3,292.05
Egg (oocyte) retrieval procedure	13212	$413.50	75% = $310.15 / 85% = $351.50
Embryo transfer	13215	$129.70	75% = $97.30 / 85% = $110.25
Preparation and transfer of a frozen or donor embryo (used instead of 13212/13215 in a frozen cycle)	13218	$949.75	75% = $712.35 / 85% = $845.25

Two things worth understanding about this table:

The monitoring ultrasounds and blood tests during your cycle are not separately billed to Medicare: they're bundled into item 13200 or 13201. That means that in practice, you won't see a string of individually rebated ultrasounds and pathology tests on your Medicare statement during stimulation, even though you're having several; they're folded into that one global fee.

The 75%/85% split depends on whether the service is provided in-hospital or out-of-hospital. Egg retrieval is usually done as day surgery (an in-hospital service), which is why it's often billed at the 75% rate rather than 85%. Embryo transfer can go either way depending on your clinic's setup.

Using the higher end of the applicable rates for a first cycle in a calendar year proceeding to a fresh embryo transfer, you're looking at somewhere around **$3,930-3,945** in core Medicare benefits, before pre-cycle consultations and testing are added on top. There's no limit on how many cycles you can claim this for across your lifetime.

The two Medicare safety nets

There are two separate Medicare safety nets on top of the rebates above that can provide significant benefits, provided that you get the timing right.

The Original Medicare Safety Net (OMSN) is the smaller, simpler one. It tracks a narrow slice of your costs: the gap between the standard 85% rebate and 100% of the schedule fee. Once that adds up to **$594.40** in a calendar year (from 1 January 2026 to 31 December 2026), Medicare bumps your rebate to 100% of the schedule fee for the rest of the year. It's automatic for individuals; couples need to register to combine costs.

The Extended Medicare Safety Net (EMSN) is the one that matters most for IVF. It tracks your *full* out-of-pocket cost: the whole gap between what your clinic charges and what Medicare pays, not just the narrow OMSN slice. Once your yearly out-of-pocket costs cross the threshold, Medicare pays back **up to 80%** of anything further you spend on out-of-hospital services for the rest of that year. For 2026 the EMSN thresholds are:

- **$2,699.10** for most people
- **$861.20** if you hold a concession card or get Family Tax Benefit Part A

A single IVF cycle often produces several thousand dollars in out-of-pocket costs on its own, so many people cross this threshold partway through their first cycle of the year. That's why a second cycle later in the same calendar year is often cheaper than the first, and why it can be worth trying to keep a full round of treatment inside one calendar year rather than letting it straddle two.

One catch: some items have a **benefit cap**, a maximum the EMSN will pay for that item, no matter how big your out-of-pocket cost is. Where a cap applies, you get whichever is lower: 80% of your cost, or the cap. Item 13212 (egg retrieval), for instance, has an EMSN cap of $88.70; item 13215 (embryo transfer) is capped at $61.40; item 13218 (frozen/donor transfer) at $888.30.

Individuals are automatically enrolled in both Medicare safety nets. **Couples are not**: you need to actively register with Services Australia so your combined costs count toward one shared threshold. Do it early, before big costs start rolling in, since past costs aren't added retroactively.

Only **out-of-hospital** costs count toward either Medicare safety net, and only costs you've paid and had verified through a claim. It should be noted that egg collection is usually done as day surgery, which is classified as **in-hospital**, and in-hospital costs don't count toward either Medicare safety net at all. They're a separate cost category, sometimes partly covered by private health insurance instead.

A quick example

Say someone has already spent $2,000 in verified out-of-pocket costs in 2026 on consultations and monitoring. They then have a $700 out-of-pocket unrelated procedure. That pushes them past the $2,699.10 EMSN threshold. From then on, for the rest of that calendar year, they get back up to 80% of further out-of-pocket costs (or the relevant cap, if lower) - which can meaningfully cut the cost of their IVF cycle as well as any further cycles in that year.

Contrast that to a person who has only spent $2,000 in out-of-pocket costs before they start their IVF cycle. Even though their IVF out-of-pocket costs would mean they end up passing the $2,699.10 EMSN threshold, because they did not reach the threshold **before** commencing their IVF cycle, they need to pay the entire out-of-pocket cost of their next treatment.

You can track whether you have met your safety net threshold by speaking to Services Australia or online via MyGov if your Medicare account is linked.

PBS medication costs

The cost of medication runs on a completely separate system from the Medicare safety nets above with different thresholds and different rules.

Most fertility medications, when prescribed by a specialist for approved treatment, are listed on the **Pharmaceutical Benefits Scheme (PBS)**, which caps what you pay per script. In 2026:

- **General patients** pay up to **$25.00** per PBS script
- **Concession card holders** pay **$7.70** per script

With the PBS, a cycle's worth of medication typically runs to a few hundred dollars in total: approximately $160-290 for general patients, less for concession card holders.

The PBS Safety Net

Just like Medicare, PBS has its own safety net, with its own threshold, tracked separately. Once your family's PBS script costs for the calendar year reach the threshold, every further script gets cheaper for the rest of the year. For 2026 the PBS safety net thresholds are:

- **$1,748.20** for general patients
- **$277.20** for concession card holders

After you cross it, general patients pay the lower concessional rate of $7.70 a script, and concession card holders pay nothing at all, for the rest of that year. Everyone with a Medicare card is automatically part of this system (there's no separate sign-up), but you do need to keep your pharmacy receipts (a Prescription Record Form, available from any pharmacy) so the spending is actually tracked. You can also combine a family's scripts onto one card to reach the threshold sooner.

Summary of Medicare and PBS safety nets

To summarise, here are the key features of each system:

Which net	What payments	2026 threshold	What you get
Original Medicare Safety Net	Small gap on specialist fees	$594.40	Rebate rises to 100% of schedule fee
Extended Medicare Safety Net	Full out-of-pocket medical costs	$2,699.10 (or $861.20 concession card holder)	80% back on further out-of-pocket costs
PBS Safety Net	Medication co-payments	$1,748.20 (or $277.20 concession card holder)	Scripts drop to $7.70, or free if concession card holder

State IVF schemes

A handful of states run their own additional schemes on top of the federal Medicare and PBS schemes:

New South Wales runs the most developed state-level support of any state. The **NSW Affordable IVF Initiative** provides a number of supports including:

- Publicly supported lower cost IVF capped at $1,000 for an IVF cycle in select clinics.

- A one-off **$2,000 Fertility Treatment Rebate** for eligible patients. This is a means tested rebate that broadly requires household income to be under $116,000, or the family has a Health Care Card, or receives Family Tax Benefit.

- A $250 rebate for pre-IVF fertility testing to offset out-of-pocket costs for an Anti-Mullerian Hormone (AMH) test, pelvic ultrasound, ovulation test or semen analysis.

- Fertility preservation support for patients with a serious medical condition.

Further up to five days of paid fertility treatment leave is available for eligible NSW public servants including teachers and nurses.

Victoria runs Australia's only fully state-funded **public fertility care program**, delivered through the Royal Women's Hospital and a growing network of satellite sites across metropolitan and regional Victoria. Treatment through this program is free, with only minor out-of-pocket costs for things like medication and some diagnostic tests. It's not open-ended, though - there's a lifetime limit of two stimulated IVF or ICSI cycles per person through the public program, and it's prioritised for people facing the biggest barriers to private care: lower-income Victorians, regional patients, and those needing fertility preservation for medical reasons (like a cancer diagnosis) or donor/altruistic surrogacy support, including LGBTIQA+ individuals and single people. Wait times from referral to first appointment currently run approximately 8-16 weeks depending on the site, and referral to actual treatment can take up to about 12 months.

Queensland has moved more recently to publicly fund reproductive treatment, currently targeted specifically at people with complex medical conditions (such as cancer) that affect fertility, alongside a state-wide fertility preservation service and counselling support for those accessing publicly funded treatment. This is narrower than Victoria's broader public program.

Western Australia, South Australia, Tasmania, the ACT, and the Northern Territory don't currently run dedicated public IVF funding programs of their own.

Practical tips for budgeting

A few things I'd suggest doing:

- **Check your state's specific schemes before you assume you're only working with the national Medicare system.** NSW and Victoria in particular offer the most support.
- **Check whether a bulk-billed or low-cost private clinic operates near you** before defaulting to a public wait list or a standard-fee clinic: it may honestly offer the best of both worlds, where available.
- **Time cycles within a calendar year where possible**, to make the most of the Extended Medicare Safety Net threshold once you've crossed it.
- **Register as a couple for both the Medicare and PBS safety nets early**, before large costs start rolling in.
- **Ask your clinic for a full written cost estimate**, not just the headline cycle fee: many costs often sit outside that number and add up, which I'll go into in more detail in the next chapter.

Chapter Seven

The Add-Ons: ICSI, PGT-A, Donor Gametes, Storage Fees and More

This is the chapter about the costs that are outside the headline cycle fee: the ones that turn a $6,000 quote into something quite different. None of what follows is automatically part of every cycle. Some of it will be medically necessary for you specifically; some of it will be offered as an option, and it really helps to understand the difference before you say yes to anything. A good specialist will explain why they're recommending something for *you*, not just that it exists.

We first cover the most common add-ons to help you build a realistic budget, followed by a discussion of less common add-ons.

ICSI (Intracytoplasmic Sperm Injection)

What it is: instead of mixing eggs and sperm together in a dish and letting fertilisation happen on its own (standard IVF), an embryologist selects a single sperm and injects it directly into each mature egg. It's commonly used where there is male-factor infertility (low sperm count, poor motility, or abnormal morphology), where natural fertilisation in a dish is unlikely to happen reliably on its own.

Cost: typically adds somewhere in the order of **$1,500-2,000** to a standard cycle, though this varies significantly by clinic.

Is it necessary for you? If your specialist has identified a male-factor issue from the semen analysis, ICSI is a truly evidence-based recommendation. Where it gets murkier is when ICSI is offered as a routine default for everyone, regardless of sperm quality, on the reasoning that it "can't hurt": the evidence for a benefit in cases without a male-factor diagnosis is actually mixed.

PGT-A (Preimplantation Genetic Testing for Aneuploidy)

What it is: a small number of cells are biopsied from a developing embryo (usually at the blastocyst stage) and tested for the correct number of chromosomes before a transfer decision is made. The idea is to identify and prioritise embryos with the best chance of implanting and developing normally, and to avoid transferring an embryo unlikely to result in a viable pregnancy.

Cost: this is often priced **per embryo**, not as one flat fee. Australian clinics typically charge somewhere in the order of **$770-950 per embryo** for the combined biopsy and genetic analysis, often with a capped maximum once you're testing a larger batch (for instance, one major provider caps the fee at seven embryos from the same egg collection). In practice, this means your actual total depends on how many embryos you have reach the stage where testing is possible: someone testing two or three embryos might pay somewhere in the **$1,500-2,800** range, while someone with a larger batch could approach **$5,000-6,500**.

There is **no Medicare rebate for PGT-A**. This should not be confused with two related tests, PGT-M and PGT-SR, used for a known single-gene condition or structural chromosome rearrangement running in a family, rather than general screening, may attract a Medicare rebate in some circumstances

Is it necessary for you? This is one of the more distinctly debated add-ons in the field. It tends to be more clearly indicated for people with a history of recurrent miscarriage, older maternal age, or multiple previous unsuccessful transfers: situations where identifying a chromosomally normal embryo has a clearer, evidence-backed rationale. For a first cycle with no particular risk factors, the evidence for it improving your overall chance of a live birth (rather than just changing which embryo gets transferred first) is more contested.

Donor gametes

Egg and sperm donation in Australia is altruistic only: donors cannot be paid for their eggs or sperm. What you pay for, as the recipient, isn't the genetic material itself, but the reasonable costs of the donation process: the donor's medical and psychological screening, their travel and appointment costs, any lost income during the process, and the clinic's program management and coordination fees. It's why Australian donor costs look nothing like the $10,000-30,000 figures often quoted for commercial donor eggs overseas.

Donor sperm is sourced through a licensed sperm bank following strict Australian screening and quarantine requirements (donated sperm is quarantined for around six months and re-tested for infectious disease before release for use). Typical cost is approximately **$500-1,500 per vial**, on top of your cycle fees.

Donor egg costs are less standardised and depend on whether you're using a known donor (someone you've arranged yourself, sometimes a friend or family member) or an unknown donor sourced through your clinic's donor program or an affiliated donor bank. Where a clinic-coordinated program is involved, expect the screening, counselling, legal, and program management costs alone to run to approximately **$3,000-6,000**, before your actual IVF cycle costs. Some clinics also partner with international donor egg banks for frozen donor oocytes shipped to Australia, which involves its own separate fee structure specific to that program.

Whether a Medicare rebate is available for donor-program treatment generally depends on there being an identified **medical reason** for needing donor gametes - if there's no medical reason on record (for instance, a single person or a same-sex couple using donor sperm by necessity of their family structure rather than a diagnosed medical condition), Medicare rebates may not apply. I cover donor conception's legal and practical side properly in Chapter Eighteen.

Storage fees

Once you have embryos, eggs, or sperm frozen, ongoing storage isn't a one-off cost: it's a **recurring fee**, charged monthly or annually, for as long as you choose to keep them stored. A typical figure is around **$40-50 per month**, charged **per gamete type** (meaning frozen embryos, frozen eggs, and frozen sperm are each billed separately if you have more than one in storage). This is always an out-of-pocket cost, and it's truly easy to lose track of as a recurring subscription-style expense once the intensity of active treatment has passed.

A practical note: if you have surplus embryos frozen after a cycle, it may be worth deciding early on a rough plan (how many cycles you might use them for, and an estimated time horizon for that decision) rather than letting storage fees quietly accumulate for years on embryos you haven't yet made an active decision about.

Bringing it together: a realistic add-on budget

None of these apply to every cycle, and it would be misleading to add them all together as if they do. But as a planning reference:

Add-on	Typical cost
ICSI	$1,500-2,000
PGT-A (per embryo, biopsy + genetic testing)	$770-950 per embryo, often capped for larger batches - typically ~$1,500-6,500 total depending on embryo count
Donor sperm	$500-1,500 per vial
Donor egg program (screening, counselling, coordination)	$3,000-6,000+
Storage (embryos, eggs, or sperm)	$40-50 per month, per gamete type

Other add-ons

Depending on your circumstances, other less common add-ons may be recommended, such as PGT-M and PGT-SR (used for screening specific, known genetic risks) and TESE (a surgical procedure to retrieve sperm directly from the testicle where ejaculation is not possible, e.g. post-vasectomy).

There are also a range of optional add-ons that could be offered to you such as:

- EmbryoGlue
- Assisted hatching
- Endometrial scratching
- Endometrial Receptivity Analysis (ERA)
- Acupuncture
- Corticosteroids (e.g. prednisolone)
- Growth hormone
- Intralipid infusions
- Immune therapies
- PICSI
- Piezo-ICSI
- Platelet-rich plasma (PRP): ovarian rejuvenation
- Platelet-rich plasma (PRP): uterine infusion
- Preimplantation Genetic Testing for Aneuploidy (PGT-A)
- Natural Killer (NK) cell testing
- Heparin

These are discussed in further detail in Chapter Sixteen. **Spoiler alert**: the current evidence on these optional add-ons and their improvements to outcomes is at best weak or non-existent.

Chapter Eight

What Private Health Insurance Covers

I've included this chapter as I know many people wonder whether paying an additional premium on their private health insurance for ART services is worth it or not.

The short of it is that private health insurance in Australia only helps with the in-hospital part of an IVF cycle. It does nothing for the out-of-hospital part. Extras cover could help with the cost of any complementary treatments that are used as part of your IVF journey; however, it doesn't assist with the costs of IVF treatment itself.

What your policy covers

Egg collection (and in limited circumstances, embryo transfer) is often done under sedation or light general anaesthetic, in an operating theatre, which makes it an in-hospital cost, even though you're usually home again within hours. These are the parts private health insurance can help with, specifically:

- **Hospital accommodation and theatre fees** for the day-surgery admission
- **A benefit toward your anaesthetist's fee**
- **A benefit toward your specialist's fee** for the procedure itself, on top of the Medicare rebate (though you may still owe a gap above what both together cover)
- **Some non-PBS medications**, if your policy has appropriate extras cover

Without insurance, the day-hospital and anaesthetist components alone typically cost somewhere in the order of **$2,000-2,800** out-of-pocket in a standard private clinic, payable on the day of admission (this varies by clinic and by which specialist day hospital is used).

Everything **out-of-hospital** (specialist consultations, monitoring ultrasounds and blood tests during stimulation, initial diagnostic testing) sits entirely outside what private health insurance covers, regardless of how good your policy is.

Does insurance cover ICSI, PGT-A, or other add-ons?

Generally, no. ICSI, PGT-A and most other add-ons are lab and embryology costs, billed directly by your clinic or an external genetics lab, not hospital-admission items.

The waiting period

Most Australian health funds treat infertility as a pre-existing condition, which means a **12-month waiting period** typically applies before your policy will pay any benefit for IVF-related hospital admissions. This starts from when you take out the policy, or from when you upgrade to a level of cover that includes ART services. If you switch to a different fund at the same level of cover, most funds will honour time you've already served; upgrading your level of cover, though, generally means serving the wait again for the newly added benefit.

One more potential wrinkle: some policies also carry a separate **benefit limitation period** (an initial window, sometimes one to three years, during which only a reduced benefit is paid for certain treatments), even after the standard waiting period has technically passed. This is honestly easy to miss in a policy document, so carefully review your policy for this carveout.

What extras cover can help with

No extras policy, however comprehensive, contributes anything toward the IVF procedure itself (except for non-PBS medications as noted above). **What extra cover can help with** is the supporting care around treatment, if your policy includes the right categories:

- **Acupuncture and Chinese medicine**, delivered by an AHPRA-registered practitioner is commonly included in mid-to-higher extras tiers, typically rebating **$15-50 per consultation**, with its own shorter waiting period (commonly two to six months).
- **Naturopathy** was stripped from standard extras cover in 2019 but became eligible again from July 2025 - funds now choose individually whether to include it.
- **Dietitian and nutritionist consultations** may be relevant if diet management is part of your approach. Commonly rebated around $45 a visit, with annual caps often starting around $200-400 depending on the fund and how long you've held the policy.
- **Exercise physiologist consultations** may be useful if PCOS or weight management is relevant.
- **Remedial massage** can help with managing the stress of the IVF process.
- **Psychology, counselling, and hypnotherapy** may also be helpful. However note that fertility counselling will already be provided by your clinic as part of treatment.

Summary

If you're even loosely anticipating that IVF might be in your future, taking out or upgrading an appropriate hospital policy now, well before you expect to need it, is the only way insurance will actually be useful when the time comes. Starting the process and taking out a policy at the same time doesn't work: you'll likely be in hospital for your first retrieval well before the 12 months is up, and get no benefit at all for it.

Chapter Nine

Budgeting and Financing More Than One Cycle

Every cost conversation is structured as if only one IVF cycle is required. However, the starting assumption, statistically, is that you'll need more than one. A realistic multi-cycle budget should include:

- **Core cycle cost after Medicare**: approximately $4,400-8,800 for a standard private clinic, or $1,000-3,000 for a low-cost/bulk-billed provider, per cycle, less any state scheme rebates
- **Private health insurance gap**: if applicable, this potentially reduces the day-hospital cost, but only if you've already served any waiting periods
- **Add-ons that apply to you**: the add-on costs listed in Chapter Seven, for example, ICSI, PGT-A, donor program costs, storage and other treatments.
- **A second and third cycle**: generally cheaper than the first if timed within the same calendar year, once you've crossed the Medicare EMSN threshold

Having regard to the above, a total of two to three cycles, for someone at a standard private clinic with no major add-ons, lands somewhere in the **$10,000-20,000** range across the full attempt, noticeably less at a low-cost provider, more if ICSI, PGT-A, or a donor program are part of your situation.

Multi-cycle package pricing

Some Australian clinics do offer discounted multi-cycle packages or bundled pricing if you commit to more than one cycle upfront. These packages are designed to provide financial certainty and may appear attractive because many patients require more than one treatment cycle before achieving a live birth.

However, it is important to understand exactly what you are purchasing before committing. Not all packages are structured the same way. Some may cover only the core IVF treatment costs, while medications, additional procedures, embryo storage, genetic testing, anaesthetist fees, donor services, or optional add-ons may still be charged separately. Some packages also have eligibility criteria, time limits, age restrictions, or conditions about the number of embryos created, cycles attempted, or circumstances in which refunds are available.

Before signing up, ask the clinic for a detailed written breakdown of what is included, what is excluded, and what happens if you achieve a pregnancy after the first cycle. Consider the package in the context of your individual circumstances, including your age, ovarian reserve, diagnosis, expected chance of success per cycle, and likelihood that you may need additional treatments.

Financing options

Even with a clear budget, financing treatment is a separate issue. A few options exist for specifically funding IVF, outside of credit cards, drawing down on your home mortgage or borrowing from friends or family.

Clinic-partnered payment plans. Several major providers (Monash IVF and others) partner with buy-now-pay-later style providers like Zip Money, typically offering 6, 12, or 24 months interest-free. This can really help spread the cost of a cycle without paying interest, but only within that window. Miss it, and the balance typically reverts to a standard variable rate (in the order of 25% p.a.), plus an ongoing account fee.

Dedicated medical finance providers. Companies like TLC Medical or MediPay offer purpose-built healthcare loans: TLC's range, for instance, runs from approximately $2,001 to $70,000 with terms up to 84 months. It's worth shopping this the way you'd shop any loan: comparing a couple of providers rather than accepting the first one your clinic suggests, since interest rates vary meaningfully between lenders.

Superannuation early release, on compassionate grounds is a commonly misunderstood option. The Australian Taxation Office (ATO) has been explicit: there is no specific compassionate-release ground for IVF treatment itself, and infertility alone isn't sufficient grounds for early release.

What may work is demonstrating that the treatment addresses a genuine, diagnosed mental health impact connected to the infertility (an "acute or chronic mental disturbance," in the ATO's language), which requires supporting reports from two registered medical practitioners, sometimes including a psychiatrist. On top of that, you generally need to show you can't reasonably afford the treatment through savings, a loan, or selling assets, and that it isn't reasonably available through the public system. You can't apply for costs you've already paid (this only works prospectively, before you spend the money), and releases are generally limited to one application per 12-month period, with no guarantee of approval. This is an option for some people, but with a real long-term cost to your retirement savings, and it deserves a conversation with a financial adviser or the ATO directly.

Part Three

The Process

Chapter Ten

How a Cycle Actually Works, Step by Step

This Part is about the logistics of IVF and how the experience actually looks like when you are going through it.

We start off in this chapter by walking through a medicated standard fresh IVF cycle from the first phone call to the pregnancy test. Several of these steps get their own deeper treatment later in this part of the book so think of this chapter as the itinerary, and those as the detailed stops along the way.

Day 1: it starts with your period

An IVF cycle officially begins on day one of your period. Most clinics ask you to call or message them on the first day of full flow, which sets everything else in motion: confirming your treatment plan, scheduling your first monitoring appointment, and making sure your medication is ready to collect. Stimulation medication itself doesn't usually start immediately (often day two or three of your cycle), but the day-one call is what triggers the whole schedule.

Before this point, you'll typically have had a planning appointment where a nurse walks you through your specific protocol, teaches you the mechanics of self-injecting, and goes through consent paperwork. Some protocols also involve a "priming" phase in the month before stimulation even starts (oral contraceptives or other hormone suppressants, used to help synchronise your cycle for treatment), though not everyone needs this step.

Stimulation: Days 2 to 12

This is the phase most people picture when they think of IVF: daily injections, usually self-administered into the lower abdomen with a very fine needle, typically lasting somewhere between 8 and 14 days. The medication (generally FSH-based, sometimes combined with other hormones depending on your specific protocol) encourages your ovaries to develop multiple follicles at once, rather than the single one a natural cycle usually produces. The aim isn't to create eggs that wouldn't otherwise exist; it's to help more of your body's existing egg-containing follicles mature in the same cycle, giving you a better chance of retrieving several viable eggs.

Throughout this phase, you'll have monitoring visits approximately every 2-3 days: a blood test and a transvaginal ultrasound scan, checking hormone levels and follicle growth. Your care team uses this to adjust your medication dose in real time and to judge when your follicles are approaching the right size for retrieval.

Mild physical and emotional side effects (bloating, cramping, breast tenderness, mood shifts, fatigue) are common during this phase as hormone levels rise.

The trigger shot

Once your lead follicles reach a mature size (generally somewhere around 17-22mm), you'll be given precise instructions for a trigger injection: a dose of hCG (sometimes combined with another medication, depending on protocol) that completes the final maturation of your eggs and sets ovulation in motion. This is timed extremely precisely: egg retrieval is scheduled for approximately 34-38 hours after the trigger, deliberately just before ovulation would naturally occur, so the eggs can be collected while still inside the follicles rather than released into the body. Getting the trigger timing right matters more than almost any other single step in the cycle, and your clinic will give you an exact time, not just a date.

Egg retrieval (day 0 of the lab process)

Egg retrieval (sometimes called an egg pick-up or EPU) is a day-surgery procedure, done under sedation or light general anaesthetic. Using ultrasound guidance, your specialist passes a fine needle through the vaginal wall into each ovary, drawing fluid from the mature follicles; the eggs are contained within that fluid. The procedure itself typically takes well under an hour, and most people go home the same day.

Your eggs are handed to the embryology lab immediately, where they're assessed for maturity. Only mature eggs are able to be fertilised.

Fertilisation: the same day

A few hours after retrieval, your eggs are fertilised - either through conventional insemination (eggs and prepared sperm placed together in a dish, allowing fertilisation to happen on its own) or ICSI (a single sperm injected directly into each mature egg), depending on what your specialist has determined is appropriate for your situation. Fertilisation is checked approximately 16-18 hours later, looking for two pronuclei: the sign that sperm and egg have meaningfully combined. You'll usually get a call with your fertilisation results by the next morning.

Embryo culture: days 1 to 5 (or 6)

From here, the fertilised eggs, now embryos, are cultured in the lab, watched as they divide: approximately 2-4 cells by day two, 6-8 cells by day three, and, for those that continue developing well, the blastocyst stage by day five or six: a much larger, more complex structure of hundreds of cells, and the point at which embryos are usually either transferred or frozen. Not every embryo that fertilises will reach blastocyst stage; this attrition is a normal, expected part of the biology.

Many clinics now use time-lapse incubators that photograph embryos continuously without disturbing them, giving embryologists a fuller picture of development without extra handling.

Embryo transfer: fresh or frozen

Two types of embryo transfers are offered:

A **fresh transfer** happens around day five after retrieval, in the same cycle: a quick, generally painless procedure where a single embryo is placed into the uterus via a thin catheter, without anaesthetic. Any additional viable embryos are frozen for possible future use.

Increasingly common, though, is a **"freeze-all" cycle**, where every viable embryo is frozen at the blastocyst stage, and the transfer happens later, in a separate frozen embryo transfer (FET) cycle. This might be recommended for several reasons: if PGT-A testing is being done and results take one to two weeks, if there's a risk of ovarian hyperstimulation syndrome (OHSS) from the stimulation phase (affecting a small percentage of cycles), or simply because your specialist judges your uterine lining will be better prepared in a subsequent, unstimulated cycle rather than the same one.

Luteal support and the wait

After a fresh transfer, you'll typically be prescribed progesterone support (often as a pessary, injection, or oral medication) to help sustain the uterine lining through the critical early days after transfer. Then comes the two-week wait: approximately nine to fourteen days, depending on your clinic's specific protocol, before a blood test (a beta hCG test) can reliably confirm whether implantation has occurred.

The overall timeline

From the start of stimulation to a fresh embryo transfer is typically around three to four weeks; adding the two-week wait brings a full fresh cycle to somewhere around five to six weeks, start to finish. If you're doing a freeze-all cycle with a separate FET, the overall timeline extends further, sometimes by several weeks to a couple of months, depending on when you and your specialist decide to proceed with the transfer.

None of these timeframes are a promise about your own cycle: bodies respond differently, protocols get adjusted mid-cycle based on how you're responding, and it's distinctly common for the exact dates to shift by a few days in either direction as your clinic fine-tunes things in real time.

Chapter Eleven

The Decisions Behind the Process

An IVF cycle isn't one continuous, predetermined sequence. It's a series of decisions, mostly made by your specialist with your input, some made in real time based on how your body is responding on the day. This chapter walks through what's being decided at each stage, what tends to drive that decision, and the terminology your clinic will use when they talk you through it.

Choosing a stimulation protocol

Before your cycle starts, your specialist chooses a protocol: the specific combination and sequence of medications used to stimulate your ovaries. This isn't one-size-fits-all, and the choice is driven by your ovarian reserve, your risk of overstimulation, and how you've responded to previous cycles, if you've had any.

The **antagonist protocol** is the most common default today. Stimulation medication (FSH) starts early in your cycle, and a second medication (an antagonist, such as Cetrotide or Orgalutran) is added partway through specifically to stop you from ovulating before retrieval. It's shorter than the alternative below, and it carries a lower risk of ovarian hyperstimulation syndrome (OHSS), which is part of why it's become the standard starting point for most patients.

The **agonist protocol** (sometimes called the "long protocol") takes a different approach: a GnRH agonist (Lucrin, Synarel, Decapeptyl) is used first to temporarily switch off your natural hormone cycle - called down-regulation - before stimulation begins at all.

This gives your clinic more complete control over timing, and it's still chosen deliberately in specific situations: endometriosis, certain patterns of poor response to the antagonist protocol, or where a clinic's own data suggests it suits your specific profile better. It takes longer and involves more medication overall, which is the trade-off for that extra control.

A **natural cycle or mini-IVF** approach uses little or no stimulation medication, working with the single egg your body would produce on its own, or a very small, mildly stimulated number. It's chosen far less often, for a specific medical reason or personal preference, and it comes with a real trade-off: lower success rates per cycle, because you're working with one egg instead of several.

The trigger decision

Near the end of stimulation, once your follicles are the right size, a **trigger shot** is given: the final injection that completes egg maturation and sets a precise 34-38 hour countdown to ovulation, timed so retrieval happens just before your body would release the eggs on its own. Most triggers are hCG-based (Ovidrel, Pregnyl). Some protocols use a **dual trigger** instead (combining hCG with a GnRH agonist), chosen specifically for patients at higher risk of OHSS, since it can lower that risk while still triggering full maturation. Which trigger you're given, and exactly when, isn't incidental: it's a decision made in real time based on how your specific cycle has responded, and the precise timing matters more than almost any other single step in the process.

Fresh transfer or freeze-all

You may go into a cycle expecting a fresh transfer and end up with a **freeze-all** instead: every viable embryo frozen, with the transfer happening later in a separate cycle. This is typically driven by one of a few things: a higher risk of OHSS, genetic testing that needs one to two weeks for results, or your specialist judging that your uterine lining will be better prepared in a subsequent, unstimulated cycle. This is one of the bigger protocol decisions made partway through a cycle, sometimes only once your bloods and scans are in.

Conventional insemination or ICSI

At fertilisation, your eggs are combined with sperm in one of two ways: **conventional insemination**, where eggs and prepared sperm are simply placed together in a dish and left to fertilise naturally, or **ICSI** (intracytoplasmic sperm injection), where an embryologist injects a single selected sperm directly into each mature egg. ICSI is the standard response to male-factor infertility (low count, poor motility, or abnormal shape) where natural fertilisation is unlikely to happen reliably in a dish. The decision point comes down to whether your specific results show a male-factor issue that makes ICSI the more reliable option.

How an embryo forms

Before the next decision makes sense, it helps to understand what's happening in the lab over the days after fertilisation.

About 16-18 hours after insemination or ICSI, embryologists check for two pronuclei (2PN): two distinct structures inside the cell, one from each parent's genetic material, and the first visible sign that fertilisation has happened. From there, the fertilised egg, now an embryo, begins to divide. By day two, it's typically split into two to four cells; by day three, six to eight: this is called the cleavage stage, while the embryo is still a small, loose cluster of individual cells. Occasionally a transfer happens at this earlier stage, though it's less common than waiting further.

Between days five and six, an embryo that's continued developing well transforms into something far more complex: a blastocyst, made up of hundreds of cells organised into two distinct groups: an inner cell mass that will go on to become the baby, and an outer layer (the trophectoderm) that will become the placenta. This is the point at which most embryos are either transferred or frozen. Not every fertilised egg reaches this stage; a meaningful number stop developing somewhere along the way, which is normal biological attrition.

Embryos frozen at this point are preserved using vitrification, a fast-freezing technique that largely replaced older, slower methods because it causes far less damage to the cell, part of why frozen embryo outcomes today are as strong as they are.

Choosing which embryo to transfer

Every blastocyst is graded by an embryologist using a shorthand like "4AA": assessing how expanded it is, the quality of the inner cell mass, and the quality of the outer cell layer. Higher grades are generally associated with better implantation potential, but grading isn't a guarantee in either direction: lower-graded embryos do result in healthy pregnancies, and higher-graded ones don't always implant. When you have more than one embryo, your clinic will almost always transfer them one at a time, in the order judged most likely to succeed based on this grading.

If you've had PGT-A genetic testing, there's a second layer added to this decision: each tested embryo comes back euploid (chromosomally normal), aneuploid (abnormal), or mosaic: a mix of normal and abnormal cells in the same embryo. Aneuploid embryos are typically not transferred as they are unlikely to result in a live birth. Mosaic results were once treated as an automatic reason to discard an embryo; that view has shifted, and many are now considered for transfer in specific circumstances with proper counselling. If genetic testing is part of your process, the decision about which embryo to transfer first is no longer just about grading - it's a conversation about grading and genetic result together, and it's worth asking your specialist to walk you through how they weigh the two if you're choosing between embryos that look different on each measure.

Banking embryos

If you have been diagnosed with diminished ovarian reserve, you may instead be offered a different strategy: embryo banking. This means doing several stimulation and retrieval cycles back to back, before attempting any transfer, to build up a pool of embryos. It's typically raised when a low AMH, a low antral follicle count, or a prior cycle with a disappointingly small egg yield suggests a single retrieval won't produce enough embryos to work with on its own, and it comes up especially often alongside PGT-A, since testing narrows an already small pool further. This is one of the bigger strategic decisions in a lower-reserve situation, and it isn't right for everyone. It takes more time, more medication, and more cost upfront, so your specialist will weigh your age, your numbers, and how urgently time matters before recommending it.

Chapter Twelve

Complementary Approaches: Diet, Exercise, Acupuncture and More

At some point in this process, someone will suggest acupuncture, supplements they heard about, or a diet overhaul. Maybe a friend, maybe a forum, maybe your own clinic.

A large Australian study found that among women with diminished ovarian reserve, 88% had been advised by someone, often outside their fertility clinic, to try complementary and integrative medicine.

All of it deserves a proper, honest look, because "some people swear by it" and "there's good evidence for it" are two very different claims.

Diet

This is the area with the most evidence behind it. A number of studies have found that following a Mediterranean-style diet (which broadly consists of vegetables, legumes, whole grains, fish, olive oil, and a modest amount of red meat) is associated with better IVF outcomes, including one widely cited study linking it to a 40% increase in pregnancy probability. It's also linked to improved semen parameters in men, including less DNA fragmentation.

Supplements are murkier. A 2024 evidence review found reasonable support for CoQ10 and DHEA, specifically for people with a history of poor ovarian response to stimulation, taken in the lead-up to a cycle. Evidence for omega-3s, melatonin, and myo-inositol (the last most relevant for PCOS) is more limited but still exists. For most other supplements marketed for fertility, the evidence is thin to absent. If you're taking anything beyond a standard pregnancy multivitamin, tell your specialist - some supplements can interact with fertility medications, and "natural" doesn't mean "without effect."

Exercise

Regular, moderate exercise (walking, swimming, gentle yoga, light strength work) is broadly supported and doesn't appear to harm outcomes; some research suggests it may modestly help, particularly for anyone managing PCOS or a higher BMI. The picture changes at the extremes. Vigorous, high-volume exercise (a commonly cited threshold is more than four hours per week of strenuous activity) has been linked in some studies to lower live birth rates and higher rates of failed implantation, thought to be related to hormonal disruption from a very high training load.

During stimulation specifically, ease off high-impact and high-intensity activity. Your ovaries are enlarged and more vulnerable to injury during this phase, and there's a real, if uncommon, risk of ovarian torsion (the ovary twisting on itself) with vigorous movement or impact. Most clinics recommend switching to walking, swimming, or gentle yoga from the start of stimulation through to your pregnancy test, then taking guidance from your specialist from there. If you're an athlete or train seriously, this is worth a specific conversation with your clinic rather than assuming your normal training load is fine to continue unchanged.

The evidence for acupuncture and other complementary therapies

Acupuncture is the best-studied complementary therapy, and even then, the evidence is mixed. Some reviews of acupuncture performed on the day of embryo transfer have found improved implantation rates; other, more recent trials have found no effect at all.

A 2026 review by the University of Melbourne's Evidence-based IVF research group (the closest thing Australia has to an independent verdict on this) found acupuncture has the strongest evidence base of any complementary therapy used in fertility care, and still describes that evidence as inconclusive.

Other complementary therapies such as naturopathy, Chinese herbal medicine, massage and meditation, have even less evidence behind them specifically for fertility outcomes. Meditation has no demonstrated effect on fertility, but it doesn't interfere with treatment either. Herbal medicine is a different matter: some preparations can interact with fertility medications or hormones, so disclose anything you're taking to your medical team.

None of this means complementary care is inherently suspect: plenty of acupuncturists, naturopaths, and dietitians work thoughtfully alongside fertility clinics, and several major providers partner with exactly these kinds of practitioners. The line worth watching for is between support offered alongside your medical care, and a promise of results the evidence doesn't back up, sold to you at a moment when you're least equipped to interrogate it critically.

Chapter Thirteen

Injections and Monitoring

If the idea of daily self-injections is the thing sitting heaviest on your chest right now, you are not being dramatic, and you're honestly not alone in this. Most people going through IVF have never given themselves an injection before in their life, and then find themselves doing it daily, sometimes twice daily, for a week or two. That's a real adjustment, phobia or not. I wanted to dedicate a chapter to injections because my fear of them was one of the key things holding me back from considering IVF at first.

The two types of injection

Almost everything in a standard stimulation protocol is a **subcutaneous** injection: delivered just under the skin, into the fatty tissue, usually in the lower abdomen. These use a very short, very fine needle, and most people find them far more manageable than they expected, often within the first day or two. The common technique: pinch or pull the skin slightly away from the muscle underneath, insert the needle at the angle your nurse showed you, and it's over in seconds. A "quick sharp pinch" is a more accurate description for most people than "painful."

A smaller number of medications (progesterone in oil is the main one) are **intramuscular**, usually given in the upper outer part of the buttock, using a longer needle. These tend to be the ones people find more uncomfortable, not because of the needle itself, but because the medication (often a thick oil) can sting going in. If you're prescribed this, ask your nurse to mark the exact spot for you the first time, and don't be shy about asking again if you're unsure.

Practical tips for injections

The following things can make a difference:

- **For subcutaneous injections**: icing the site for 15-30 seconds beforehand meaningfully dulls the surface nerves enough to blunt the sensation. Pinching the skin firmly (not so hard you bruise) also helps distract from the pinch of entry.

- **For intramuscular injections**: counterintuitively, ice isn't the answer here. A warm compress or heating pad for 5-10 minutes beforehand relaxes the muscle and can make the injection more comfortable, and warming the medication itself (for example, using your hands or a warm water bath) can reduce the sting of a cold, thick oil going in.

- **Numbing cream**: a topical anaesthetic (lidocaine-based, or the prescription option Emla) applied approximately 30-45 minutes before an injection can take the edge off considerably. It won't remove all sensation, but if you have needle anxiety ask your nurse coordinator whether they can prescribe or recommend one.

- **Rotate your injection sites**: alternating sides and slightly different spots on the abdomen reduces soreness building up in one area over a week or two of daily injections.

- **Let alcohol swabs dry fully** before injecting: this alone prevents a surprising amount of unnecessary stinging.

- **Have a simple, consistent routine**: same time of day, same clean, well-lit space, medications and sharps container laid out before you start.

Some people find self-injecting easier, because there's no waiting for someone else to work up the nerve, and you're fully in control of the timing and technique. Others find it much easier to have a partner, friend, or family member do it, because it removes the mental step of having to be the one to actually push the needle in. If you have a partner involved in this process, discuss early who will do this and how.

If someone else is doing the injecting for you, it's worth both of you attending the nurse teaching session together, or having them watch instruction videos on how to inject the medication correctly until they're comfortable.

If this is a phobia, not just nerves

There's a real, meaningful difference between finding injections unpleasant and having a needle phobia: the kind that causes real panic, fainting, or avoidance behaviour. If that's you, please say so early to your clinic. This is something fertility nurses have supported people through many times before, and there are real, practical options:

- **Cognitive behavioural therapy (CBT)** is a well-established, evidence-based treatment specifically for needle and medical phobias, and some people find even a short course of sessions really changes their experience of the whole process, not just the injections.

- **Structured desensitisation** with your nurse coordinator: practising the mechanics slowly, with support, before you're doing it under time pressure at home.

- **Full delegation** to a partner or support person, with you not required to watch or handle the needle at all, if that's what truly works for you.

None of these are a lesser path than "toughing it out." A good clinic will treat this request the same way they'd treat any other clinical concern.

Dealing with bruising

Bruising is one of the most common, and obvious, side effects of injections. The bruising tends to worsen as a cycle progresses, partly because you are cycling through a limited area of skin and partly because some of the medications (and the blood-thinning medication some people are prescribed alongside them) can make capillaries more prone to leaking. Rotating injection sites, applying gentle ice before and warmth after, and injecting slowly can all reduce bruising. For most, it's a manageable nuisance rather than a medical concern, though larger bruises, significant swelling, or pain warrant a call to the clinic to rule out issues like an infection or a missed subcutaneous injection that went into muscle.

Monitoring: the other needles

Along with the injections themselves, the monitoring visits during stimulation involve their own blood draws, approximately every two to three days. If needles are a source of anxiety generally, flag this to the nursing team too. Many clinics can use a smaller butterfly needle for blood draws, or offer numbing cream here as well if you ask.

Other injection logistics

A few smaller things to consider around injections:

- **Check storage requirements for each medication as soon as you collect it**: some need refrigeration, others don't, and mixing this up can affect the medication.

- **Sharps disposal**: your clinic or pharmacy will provide a proper sharps container; never dispose of needles in household rubbish. Most clinics or local councils offer a return or collection service; ask your nurse coordinator what's available in your area.

- **Travelling during stimulation**: if you need to travel during your injection window, ask in advance about safely transporting medication (an insulated bag for anything needing refrigeration) and whether your clinic can advise on timing flexibility if your schedule shifts.

Chapter Fourteen

Egg Retrieval and Embryo Transfer

This chapter is about two of the most critical days in an IVF cycle: the egg retrieval and the embryo transfer. We'll cover the practical, physical and slightly mundane details of what those two days look like.

Egg retrieval: the day itself

Before you arrive: depending on the type of anaesthetic you are using, you'll be given fasting instructions which typically means no food or drink, including water, for around 6-8 hours before the procedure. You'll need to organize for someone to drive you home and, ideally, stay with you for the rest of the day.

Local anaesthetic involves numbing the vaginal wall with a local anaesthetic while you remain fully awake. It has the shortest recovery time but may be less comfortable, particularly if many eggs are expected to be collected. Some people also prefer this option as it allows them to discuss egg numbers with their medical team as the egg collection is occurring.

Twilight sedation (intravenous sedation) is the most common approach in Australia. Sedative and pain-relieving medications are given through a drip to make you relaxed and sleepy, with little or no memory of the procedure, while you continue breathing on your own.

General anaesthesia puts you into a deeper state of unconsciousness for the procedure and may be recommended in some situations, such as complex egg retrievals or where clinically appropriate.

Your fertility specialist and anaesthetist will recommend the most suitable option based on your medical history, the planned procedure and your clinic's usual practice.

A practical packing list: loose, comfortable clothing that won't put pressure on your abdomen, a water bottle, a small snack for after, sanitary pads, and something to occupy yourself during the recovery wait - a podcast, book, music, or simply company if your support person is allowed to stay nearby.

What actually happens: once you're in the procedure room, you'll be connected to monitoring equipment, and your anaesthetist (if required) will talk you through what to expect before you're sedated. Using the same transvaginal ultrasound probe used for your monitoring scans, now fitted with a fine needle guide, your specialist passes a needle through the vaginal wall into each ovary, drawing fluid from the mature follicles. This fluid (containing the eggs, though they're microscopic and not visible to the naked eye) is immediately handed to the embryology lab next door, where the eggs are identified under a microscope. The whole procedure typically takes somewhere between 15 and 30 minutes. On average, somewhere between 8 and 15 eggs are collected, though this varies enormously by age, ovarian reserve, and how you responded to stimulation.

Waking up and recovery: you'll wake in a recovery bay, likely feeling groggy if you've been under sedation, and be monitored for one to a few hours as the anaesthetic wears off. As it does, mild to moderate cramping, similar to a bad period, is common; clinics typically offer pain relief and a heat pack for the abdomen. Some nausea is also common. You'll usually be given a light snack once you're properly awake, and most people are discharged within two to three hours of the procedure ending.

What to expect over the following days: some spotting or light bleeding from the puncture site is normal for a few days. Avoid tampons for about a week, to let the internal puncture site heal: pads are fine, and clinics will usually have some on hand if you need them. Bloating and mild cramping can continue for several days as your ovaries (still enlarged from stimulation) settle back down. Avoid heavy lifting or high-impact exercise for the following week or so, mainly to protect your ovaries while they're still enlarged. Many people take the rest of the day and sometimes the following day off work; others feel ready sooner.

Your clinic should flag the risk of ovarian hyperstimulation syndrome (OHSS). It happens when the ovaries respond more strongly to stimulation medication than intended, causing them to swell and, in more significant cases, fluid to leak into the abdomen.

The typical cause of OHSS is the trigger shot. The trigger shot's job is to make the eggs ready for collection. In a natural cycle, the body would do this with a surge of its own hormone (LH), but IVF uses a substitute called hCG instead, because it does the same job but stays active in the body for longer. That longer-lasting effect is exactly what makes it capable of triggering OHSS. With so many follicles growing at once (the whole aim of stimulation), the ovaries have far more hormone-producing tissue than in a natural cycle, and the hCG trigger switches all of that tissue on at the same time.

Mild symptoms of OHSS are common: some degree of bloating, abdominal discomfort, and mild nausea affects a meaningful proportion of people during a stimulated cycle, and on their own, these mild symptoms are considered a normal part of the process rather than a medical emergency.

Moderate to more significant OHSS is less common but real, occurring in approximately 1 to 5 in every 100 treatment cycles, more frequently in people with PCOS. Symptoms usually begin within a week of the trigger injection (the final shot before egg collection) and typically resolve within one to two weeks on their own. If pregnancy occurs, however, rising hCG can cause symptoms to persist and sometimes intensify for several more weeks, gradually resolving as the pregnancy progresses.

Contact your clinic's nurse line if you experience:

- Rapid abdominal bloating or a feeling of significant fullness that's worsening
- Rapid weight gain (more than approximately one kilogram in 24 hours)
- Persistent or worsening nausea and vomiting
- Reduced urination

Seek urgent medical attention (call your clinic's emergency line, or present to an emergency department if you can't reach them) if you experience:

- Severe or worsening abdominal pain
- Shortness of breath or difficulty breathing
- Inability to keep fluids down

- Significant dizziness or fainting
- Calf pain or swelling (a possible sign of a blood clot, a rare but serious complication)

Every clinic will give you their own specific after-hours contact information for exactly this reason. Save that number in your contacts so you'll actually find it under stress rather than sifting through emails in a panic.

Embryo transfer: a different kind of day

This is a completely different experience from retrieval and feels surprisingly uneventful due to how quick it is, even though it is arguably the most significant day of the entire process.

Before you arrive: unlike retrieval, there's generally no fasting requirement, since anaesthesia isn't usually involved. Most clinics will ask you to arrive with a full bladder as it helps position the uterus to make it far more visible on the ultrasound used to guide the transfer.

What actually happens: you're fully awake throughout, and most clinics allow a partner or support person into the room with you. The embryology team confirms your identity: often more than once, matching your name and date of birth against the embryo being used. A speculum is inserted (similar sensation to a pap smear), and under ultrasound guidance, your specialist threads a thin, flexible catheter containing your embryo through the cervix and releases it into the uterus. The procedure itself is generally described as painless, or close to it, and takes around 20-30 minutes including preparation: the actual embryo placement itself is much quicker than that.

Immediately after: you can empty your bladder right away and there's no medical need to lie flat or rest immediately afterward, though plenty of clinics will still let you rest in the room for a short while if you'd like to. You're able to drive yourself home, since no sedation is involved.

In the days following: most clinics recommend light activity rather than strict bed rest, avoiding high-impact exercise, hot tubs or baths (showers are fine), and intercourse until after your pregnancy test. Mild cramping or light spotting in the days after transfer is common and doesn't necessarily mean anything either way about the outcome.

Chapter Fifteen

The Two-Week Wait

The two-week wait (also known as the TWW) is the stretch between embryo transfer and the blood test that gives a reliable answer. It has a reputation, and it's earned: almost everyone who's been through it describes it as one of the hardest parts of the whole process, harder in some ways than the physical parts, because there's simply nothing to do but wait.

It's tempting to try to stay relentlessly positive, as if a negative thought might somehow affect the outcome, but trying to suppress difficult feelings usually just adds a second layer of effort on top of an already hard two weeks. It's alright to think about what a negative result would mean, to feel some grief in advance of a possibility, and to let that coexist with hope.

Why it's two weeks

Your trigger shot uses hCG (the same hormone a pregnancy test detects), which means there's already hCG in your system after transfer, left over from the trigger itself, not necessarily from a pregnancy. It takes approximately ten days for that residual hCG to clear your body completely. Test before then, and you risk a false positive from the trigger shot's leftover trace, not an actual pregnancy result. The blood test at day 10-14 is timed specifically so any hCG detected at that point can only be coming from a genuine, developing pregnancy - which is also why a blood test (measuring an exact hormone level) is more reliable than a home urine test at this stage, and why your clinic will usually ask you to hold off on home testing until they've called you with the blood result.

The symptom trap

Here's something that might cause you a huge amount of unnecessary anguish during this window: almost every symptom you might notice during the two-week wait can be explained by the progesterone support you're already taking, not by pregnancy. Breast tenderness, cramping, bloating, fatigue, mood swings, mild nausea - these are also just what progesterone does. There is no reliable way to tell, from how you feel, whether a cycle has worked. Cramping doesn't mean it hasn't worked. The absence of any symptoms doesn't mean it hasn't worked either: plenty of people who go on to have a successful pregnancy report feeling nothing unusual at all during this window.

Symptom-spotting is one of the most common ways people put themselves through unnecessary extra distress during these two weeks. If you catch yourself spiraling, try and distract yourself or speak to someone about it, including a professional where necessary.

Tips for managing the two-week wait

- **Distraction with intention**: hobbies, light outings, things that occupy your mind without requiring you to pretend nothing is happening. There's a difference between healthy distraction and trying to white-knuckle your way through by ignoring the whole situation.
- **Lean on your support people**: partner, family, friends, your clinic's fertility counsellors, or online communities. You don't have to carry this stretch alone.
- **Mind-body practices**: meditation, gentle yoga, journaling, or simply conscious breathing are commonly recommended by fertility counselling teams, not because they influence the outcome, but because they can ease the day-to-day experience of an anxious stretch of time.
- **Avoid home testing before your clinic's recommended date**, for the hCG-clearance reason above: an early test is more likely to mislead you than inform you.
- **Keep your clinic's after-hours number somewhere accessible**, if you experience significant pain, heavy bleeding, or emotional distress that feels like more than you can manage.

Chapter Sixteen

When a Cycle Doesn't Work: What Happens Next

Part Four covers the emotional weight of loss properly and at the length it deserves. This chapter is deliberately about the logistics, so that thread doesn't get tangled up with everything else you're feeling in the moment.

What a negative result means

A negative beta hCG test means implantation didn't happen, or didn't continue. It's one to keep in mind that a cycle can fail at more than one possible point: the embryo may not have implanted at all, or it may have implanted briefly and stopped developing (sometimes showing as a very brief, low positive before a negative confirms it). One unsuccessful cycle doesn't predict what a future one will do. Outcomes vary cycle to cycle depending on egg and embryo quality, the uterine environment, and a fair amount that current medicine still can't fully explain - statistically, most people need more than one attempt before a live birth.

Most people experience something like a period within approximately two weeks of a negative result, as the hormonal support is stopped and the uterine lining sheds. This can come with its own cramping and emotional weight, layered on top of everything else. Mention it to your clinic if it feels unusually heavy, prolonged, or painful.

What the next appointment looks like

Most clinics won't rush you into a detailed review conversation immediately, for good reason. The immediate aftermath of a negative result is not usually the moment for a clear-headed conversation about next steps, and a good clinic will let the initial shock settle before booking that appointment, generally within the following one or two weeks.

The review appointment is where your specialist looks back over the specific details of your cycle to identify whether the plan should be repeated as-is or adjusted. Depending on where things didn't go as hoped, this might include:

- **Ovarian response** - how many eggs were retrieved and matured, and whether the stimulation protocol or dosing should be adjusted for a future cycle

- **Fertilisation and embryo development** - how many eggs fertilised, how far embryos developed, and whether ICSI or other lab techniques might change for next time

- **Embryo quality and grading**, and whether PGT-A might be worth considering if it wasn't already used

- **The uterine environment** - whether the endometrial lining looked receptive, and whether anything about timing or preparation should change

For most people, after a single unsuccessful cycle, this review is enough to inform a next attempt without further testing. One cycle not working is common and shouldn't be taken to automatically mean that something is fundamentally wrong.

When further investigation becomes relevant

If you've had two or more cycles with good-quality embryos that haven't resulted in a pregnancy, this is sometimes referred to as recurrent implantation failure. Further investigation may be warranted at this stage rather than repeating the same protocol again. This might include a closer look at the uterine cavity (sometimes a hysteroscopy: a procedure to examine inside the uterus, which some research suggests can modestly improve outcomes in a subsequent cycle for people in this situation), testing for chronic endometritis (a subtle, often symptom-free inflammation of the uterine lining that's been increasingly recognised as a contributing factor in some cases), or a broader review of immunological or other less common factors. This is a still-evolving area of fertility medicine, and not every proposed test or treatment in this space has equally strong evidence behind it.

Add-ons you might be offered

Beyond ICSI and PGT-A (discussed earlier in this book), you may also be offered a handful of other optional extras where you have had one or more failed cycles previously. Australian research puts this in real perspective: more than 80% of Australian IVF patients use at least one add-on, often paying thousands of dollars extra. Concerningly, a major independent evidence review in 2026 found that most of them lack good-quality evidence that they actually improve the chance of a live birth.

Australian research group Evidence-based IVF (run out of the University of Melbourne) maintains an independent, non-commercial summary of the evidence for each of these, summarised below:

EmbryoGlue

What it is: A transfer medium containing hyaluronic acid, a substance naturally found in the reproductive tract and thought to help embryos implant.

What the evidence says: One of the few add-ons with any positive signal. The 2026 review found weak evidence it may increase pregnancy and live birth rates, but the benefit isn't strong enough to be considered proven.

Cost / considerations: Usually adds a modest cost to embryo transfer. No known additional risks.

Assisted hatching

What it is: A laser is used to thin the embryo's outer shell (zona pellucida) to make it easier for the embryo to "hatch" and implant. Often offered to women over 38 or after failed IVF cycles.

What the evidence says: May improve pregnancy rates, but has not been shown to improve live birth rates. Some studies found a higher miscarriage rate, potentially cancelling out any early benefit.

Cost / considerations: Typically costs a few hundred dollars.

Endometrial scratching

What it is: A minor procedure that intentionally irritates the uterine lining before IVF, aiming to trigger an inflammatory response that improves implantation.

What the evidence says: Early studies were promising, but a large trial of more than 1,300 women found no improvement in live birth rates. The 2026 review found only weak evidence of possible benefit.

Cost / considerations: Usually performed in the cycle before IVF and involves an additional procedure.

ERA (Endometrial Receptivity Analysis)

What it is: A biopsy-based genetic test that analyses the uterine lining to identify your personal "window of implantation" so embryo transfer can be timed accordingly.

What the evidence says: Despite the appealing theory, studies have found no convincing improvement in live birth rates for most IVF patients.

Cost / considerations: Typically costs around $1,000-2,000 and requires a biopsy and an additional mock cycle.

Acupuncture

What it is: Needle therapy performed before or around embryo transfer, intended to improve uterine blood flow, reduce stress and enhance implantation.

What the evidence says: High-quality studies show no evidence that it improves pregnancy or live birth rates. Some people still choose it for relaxation or stress reduction.

Cost / considerations: Usually self-funded (unless covered by private health insurance) with little medical risk when performed by qualified practitioners.

Corticosteroids (e.g. prednisolone)

What it is: Steroid medication used to suppress the immune system, based on the theory that immune activity may interfere with implantation.

What the evidence says: Studies show no improvement in pregnancy or live birth rates for routine IVF patients.

Cost / considerations: Can cause side effects including mood changes, increased blood sugar and infection risk.

Growth hormone

What it is: Hormone injections sometimes offered to women with poor ovarian reserve or previous poor response to IVF stimulation, aiming to improve egg quality.

What the evidence says: Evidence remains inconsistent and low quality, with no reliable proof that it improves live birth rates.

Cost / considerations: One of the more expensive add-ons, often costing over $1,000 per cycle.

Intralipid infusions

What it is: An intravenous fat emulsion originally developed for hospital nutrition, repurposed to suppress immune activity that may affect implantation.

What the evidence says: Current evidence shows no convincing improvement in live birth rates, and major fertility organisations do not recommend routine use.

Cost / considerations: Requires IV treatment and adds significant cost without proven benefit.

Immune therapies

What it is: Includes treatments such as IVIG, immune-modulating drugs and therapies guided by immune testing, offered for recurrent implantation failure or miscarriage.

What the evidence says: The underlying theories remain controversial and there is no strong evidence these treatments improve live birth rates for most IVF patients.

Cost / considerations: Often very expensive and some treatments carry significant side effects.

PICSI

What it is: A variation of ICSI where sperm are selected based on their ability to bind to hyaluronic acid, with the aim of choosing more mature sperm.

What the evidence says: Has not been shown to improve pregnancy or live birth rates, although some studies suggest it may reduce miscarriage.

Cost / considerations: Usually an optional laboratory add-on at extra cost.

Piezo-ICSI

What it is: A newer form of ICSI using piezoelectric pulses to inject sperm into the egg more gently than standard ICSI.

What the evidence says: There are too few high-quality studies to determine whether it improves pregnancy or live birth rates.

Cost / considerations: Availability varies between clinics and generally incurs additional fees.

PRP (ovarian rejuvenation)

What it is: Platelet-rich plasma prepared from your own blood is injected into the ovaries in an attempt to stimulate egg production or improve ovarian function.

What the evidence says: Currently no convincing evidence that it improves live birth rates. Most experts consider it experimental.

Cost / considerations: Expensive, invasive and not routinely recommended.

PRP (uterine infusion)

What it is: Platelet-rich plasma is infused into the uterus before embryo transfer to encourage the uterine lining to thicken and become more receptive.

What the evidence says: Evidence is limited and inconclusive, with no reliable proof that it improves the chance of taking home a baby.

Cost / considerations: Usually offered to women with thin endometrium at additional cost.

PGT-A

What it is: Embryos are biopsied and tested for chromosomal abnormalities before transfer to identify those most likely to implant successfully.

What the evidence says: May reduce miscarriage and avoid transferring embryos with chromosome abnormalities, but has not consistently been shown to increase overall live birth rates per IVF cycle started. Best suited to selected patients rather than routine use.

Cost / considerations: One of the most expensive add-ons, often costing several thousand dollars.

NK cell testing

What it is: A blood or uterine test measuring natural killer (NK) cells, based on the theory that abnormal immune activity may prevent implantation.

What the evidence says: There is no agreed definition of an abnormal result, and testing has not been shown to improve IVF outcomes. Most professional organisations do not recommend routine testing.

Cost / considerations: Often leads to additional immune treatments that also lack strong evidence.

Heparin

What it is: A blood-thinning medication prescribed to improve blood flow or reduce microscopic clotting around the embryo.

What the evidence says: Beneficial for women with specific clotting disorders (such as antiphospholipid syndrome), but no convincing evidence it improves live birth rates for routine IVF patients.

Cost / considerations: Requires daily injections and carries risks including bruising and bleeding.

None of this means these add-ons are dishonest or that clinics offering them are acting in bad faith - several are offered because a patient specifically asks, or because a clinic wants to offer every reasonable option to someone who's had a difficult run. But "available" and "proven to help" are different things, and it's a fair question to ask your specialist directly: for my specific situation, is there real evidence this will change my outcome, or is this being offered as an option rather than a recommendation?

It should also be noted that IVF isn't a finished technology. It has been quietly evolving for almost 50 years and significant research is currently going into making IVF more personalised, more comfortable and more successful. You may find that new technologies and methodologies are offered to you beyond what is mentioned above.

When to consider changing clinics

Changing IVF clinics can feel like a major decision, particularly after investing time, money and emotional energy in treatment. However, you are not committed to staying with a clinic simply because you started there. It may be worth considering a change if you feel your concerns are being dismissed, communication is consistently poor, you are not receiving clear explanations about your treatment plan, or you have lost confidence in the care you are receiving. You may also want to seek a second opinion after unsuccessful treatment, particularly if you would like another specialist to review your history and discuss whether a different approach may be appropriate. A different clinic cannot guarantee a better outcome, so consider both the potential benefits and the practical costs of changing.

Before making the switch, ask both clinics about the costs and practicalities of transferring your care. If you have frozen embryos, eggs or sperm, transporting them between clinics requires coordination between the sending and receiving clinics and may involve transport, administrative or storage-related fees. You may also need to pay for a new specialist consultation or obtain copies of your medical records. Fees and procedures vary between clinics, so check the specific requirements with both providers. Ultimately, you should feel that your questions are welcomed, your options are clearly explained and you have confidence in the team providing your care.

Deciding what happens next

This is your decision, informed by your specialist's clinical read of what happened, but not dictated by it. A few things worth weighing:

- **Do you have frozen embryos already**, meaning the next step might be a frozen embryo transfer rather than a full new stimulation cycle: generally a lower-intensity, lower-cost next attempt than starting again from scratch

- **Does the review suggest a specific, targeted change**, or would a repeat of the same protocol be reasonable

- **Where are you against the cycle-count and budget conversation** you had with yourself, or with your partner: has this result changed that calculation, or does the original plan still hold

- **Do you need more time before deciding anything**? Sometimes time alone gives you the space you need to work through all the emotions and the facts before arriving at the decision that is best for you.

Chapter Seventeen

Frozen Embryo Transfers and Subsequent Cycles

A frozen embryo transfer (FET) uses an embryo that was frozen during a previous cycle (via vitrification), thawed and transferred in a separate, later cycle. No egg collection, no fertilisation, no embryo culture involved this time around; the lab work has already happened. What this cycle is really about is preparing your uterus to receive the embryo, on its own timeline, separate from any ovarian stimulation.

One reason fresh transfers were traditionally preferred to FETs was the risk of a frozen embryo not surviving the thaw. However, modern vitrification has a high survival rate - commonly cited around 95%, sometimes higher for blastocysts frozen at good quality. It's not zero risk, but it's no longer the significant point of attrition it once was with older, slower freezing methods.

Natural versus medicated: the two ways to prepare

Natural cycle FET works with your own ovulation. Your clinic monitors you with ultrasound and bloodwork through the first half of your cycle, and once your body naturally ovulates (sometimes confirmed with an hCG trigger to pin down the exact timing), the transfer is scheduled a set number of days later, matched to your embryo's stage. This only works if you're ovulating regularly and predictably.

Medicated (artificial) cycle FET uses estrogen, usually for 10-14 days, to build the uterine lining, followed by progesterone once the lining is ready, with the transfer scheduled on a specific day of progesterone exposure. This gives your clinic much tighter control over timing: useful for scheduling, and the only real option if your cycles aren't regular enough to predict naturally.

Which is better? Based on the evidence, the answer is that they produce broadly similar pregnancy outcomes for people with regular cycles, so the choice often comes down to practical preference. Medicated cycles are easier to schedule precisely (useful if you're coordinating around work, travel, or a specific timeframe) and avoid the natural cycle's unpredictability. However, natural cycles avoid the additional medication load and cost.

There's a growing body of research suggesting medicated ("programmed") FET cycles may carry a somewhat higher risk of certain pregnancy complications, including pre-eclampsia, compared with natural cycles, thought to be related to the corpus luteum (a structure formed after natural ovulation, absent in a fully medicated cycle) playing a role beyond just hormone support. This is a still-active area of research but it may be worth raising with your specialist as part of deciding which protocol suits you, particularly if you have other risk factors for pregnancy complications already.

Are there still injections?

Fewer, usually, but not necessarily zero.

The big daily FSH stimulation injections are gone entirely: that's the main injection burden of a fresh cycle, and a FET doesn't need it at all, since there's no egg collection involved. What's left depends on your specific protocol:

- **Progesterone support**, needed in both natural and medicated FET to sustain the uterine lining after transfer, is often given as a vaginal pessary or gel rather than an injection - but some clinics or specific situations use intramuscular progesterone injections instead.

- **Estrogen**, in a medicated cycle, is usually oral tablets or a skin patch, though an injectable form exists and is sometimes used.

- **A trigger shot** is sometimes still used even in a natural cycle FET, to pin down the exact timing of ovulation, so even the lowest-medication option can still involve at least one injection.

Someone on a natural cycle with a vaginal progesterone pessary might have no injections at all. Someone on a medicated cycle with intramuscular progesterone could still be injecting daily for a couple of weeks.

How FET success rates compare to fresh transfers

This tends to surprise people: several large studies have found FET success rates to be as good as, and in some populations noticeably better than, fresh transfers, plausibly because a fresh cycle's high hormone levels from stimulation can make the uterine lining less receptive than it would be in an unstimulated, later cycle. This is part of why freeze-all cycles have become increasingly common as a deliberate strategy, not just a fallback when a fresh transfer isn't possible.

How many embryos to thaw

Almost always, clinics thaw and transfer one embryo at a time, in the order judged most likely to succeed based on grading and, if you've had PGT-A testing, genetic results. This is a conversation good to have with your specialist in advance - which embryo is being used, and why, and what the plan is for the ones still in storage if this attempt doesn't work.

On timing

There's no universal rule for how soon after a fresh cycle (or a negative result) a FET should happen. Some research suggests outcomes aren't harmed, and may even be somewhat better, when there's a reasonable gap rather than the very next cycle, though this is not a strong enough basis to treat as a firm recommendation for your own timing. Practically, this means there's no evidence-based reason to feel pressured into rushing straight into a FET the moment you're medically cleared, if you need more time before starting again.

Chapter Eighteen

Donor Conception and Surrogacy

In this chapter, we'll cover the basics of donor conception, and then break out into what's specific to single women starting with donor sperm (single mothers by choice, also known as a SMBC) and LGBTQ+ issues. We'll also briefly discuss surrogacy and how that looks like in Australia as well as internationally.

The donor conception basics

Anonymous donation doesn't exist in Australia and has been banned since 2006. This surprises people used to how donor conception is portrayed overseas. Every donor (sperm, egg, or embryo) consents in advance to their identifying information such as their name, date of birth and contact details being released to any person born from their donation once that person turns 18, sometimes earlier with counsellor or parental consent. If an overseas anonymous arrangement appeals to you because it seems simpler, understand the real, lasting cost: a child conceived that way may never be able to access genetic or medical information later.

A known donor, such as a friend, or someone you've found and arranged directly, offers a real relationship and more information than a profile ever could, but carries legal complexity which is discussed further below. Independent legal advice plus a written donor agreement *before* conceiving is strongly recommended by fertility lawyers who work in this space, for everyone's protection.

A de-identified donor, sourced through a licensed clinic or sperm bank, is the more common route. Donors are screened for medical and family history, complete a detailed questionnaire (such as their interests, occupation, education, existing children), and consent in advance to the identity release described above.

A word of caution: informal donor arrangements found through online forums or social platforms, outside a licensed clinic, carry real risk. Donors aren't screened for infectious disease or genetic conditions, family-limit rules aren't tracked, and there have been documented cases of pressure toward natural rather than clinical insemination. Clinics warn against this route, and that warning is worth taking seriously even when the formal system feels frustratingly slow.

Each state in Australia with donor conception legislation keeps its own central register of donors, recipients, and donor-conceived children. There's currently no single national register.

Family limits. Most states cap how many families a single donor can be connected to. Based on current law, New South Wales and Western Australia legislate a five-family cap per donor, while Victoria, South Australia and Queensland allow up to ten. The ACT allows a five-family cap in the ACT and ten families nationally. Tasmania and the Northern Territory have no specific legislation, leaving limits to individual clinics under national NHMRC guidelines. Some jurisdictions count the donor's own family within that limit, and New South Wales recently confirmed its five-family cap applies worldwide, not just within the state. How the family limit applies to same-sex couples differs by state as well. For example, Victoria amended its law in 2021 to explicitly allow women in a same-sex relationship to use the same donor for a second child even once the state's ten-family limit is otherwise reached, treating the couple as one family throughout.

The legal position of a donor. A donor who has properly consented through a registered clinic is not a legal parent. This is exactly why informal, non-clinic arrangements are risky: outside a documented, clinic-mediated process, this legal protection isn't reliably in place.

Sourcing donor material overseas generally requires formal state approval before it can be used here, with the same consent and identity-release requirements regardless of where the donor is based. This is an administrative step that should be raised with your clinic early to avoid delaying the process, on top of the cost considerations discussed earlier.

If you're building this alone

If you're considering, or already pursuing, parenthood on your own, you're part of a growing, increasingly visible group in Australia. Testing, timelines, and the specialist pathway are the same as anyone else's. The difference shows up once you're with a specialist: for most single women on this path, the conversation moves fairly quickly to donor sperm, since that's what's standing between you and conception, not necessarily an underlying fertility issue (though it's still good to have your own fertility properly assessed, since age and reserve affect your timeline here too). Being single also doesn't change your access to a Medicare rebated cycle.

The legal landscape is still a bit unsettled. Section 60H of the Family Law Act 1975 addresses parentage for children conceived through assisted reproduction, but it was largely written with heterosexual couples in mind and doesn't offer the same explicit clarity for solo mothers, particularly with known donors. In practice, the risk of a known donor successfully claiming legal parental status is considered small. However, small isn't zero, which is exactly why a written agreement and legal advice before conception matters so much. Donor conception laws also vary by state, particularly around counselling requirements, so check your specific state's rules. Every state with legislation here requires mandatory counselling before treatment with an ANZICA-accredited counsellor.

Solo Mums by Choice Australia is a dedicated support community for women pursuing this path. It's worth seeking out specifically if you're in that boat, since general fertility communities often default to couple-centric framing.

If you're LGBTQ+

There's no single pathway here either, because there's no single starting point: a lesbian couple, a gay male couple, a bisexual or queer person, trans and non-binary people all arrive with different practical questions. This section tries to give each of these situations the specific attention it deserves.

Medicare eligibility now stands on equal footing. Until recently, Medicare's definition of infertility assumed a heterosexual couple, effectively excluding same-sex couples and single people from rebates unless they could point to a diagnosed medical condition separate from their family structure. That changed with a formal update to Medicare's eligibility rules in April 2025, extending rebate eligibility to same-sex couples and single people on the same basis as anyone else. The one real exception: this doesn't extend to surrogacy.

For lesbian and queer women, it's not unusual in these circumstances to have **reciprocal IVF** (also called co-IVF), where one partner's eggs create embryos with donor sperm and the other partner carries the pregnancy, resulting in a genetic connection for one and a gestational connection for the other.

For gay men, and anyone needing a gestational pathway: surrogacy. The domestic legal process is covered in its own section below, followed by a section on overseas pathways if that's the direction you're considering.

For trans and non-binary people, if fertility preservation matters to you (before starting gender-affirming hormone therapy, for instance) Chapter Nineteen covers this properly. Beyond preservation, the pathways above apply based on your reproductive anatomy and family-building goals, not your gender identity.

When choosing a specialist and clinic, comfort and fluency with reciprocal IVF, surrogacy coordination, or simply not defaulting to heteronormative assumptions makes a real difference to how supported you feel through a long process. Several major providers run dedicated LGBTQ+ family programs.

Rainbow Families is a dedicated advocacy and support organisation for LGBTQ+ family-building. It's a good place for both current policy information and community connection.

Surrogacy in Australia

Only altruistic surrogacy is legal in Australia, whereby a surrogate can be reimbursed for reasonable expenses but not paid for carrying the pregnancy.

Commercial surrogacy is illegal nationally, and several states apply this extraterritorially. That is, entering a commercial arrangement overseas can carry criminal liability under some state laws even though it happens abroad. At the time of writing, New South Wales, Queensland, and the Australian Capital Territory (ACT) prohibit their residents from accessing surrogacy overseas. If an overseas pathway is on your mind, engaging a lawyer who specialises specifically in Australian surrogacy law isn't optional caution, it's essential.

Western Australia currently restricts altruistic surrogacy to opposite-sex couples and requires proof of medical infertility to access IVF at all. It is the last state in the country with either restriction still in place. Reform legislation passed WA Parliament in December 2025 and will extend access to same-sex couples, single people, and transgender and intersex West Australians, while also removing the infertility requirement. However, it isn't expected to commence until mid-2027, following an 18-month implementation period during which supporting regulations are still being drafted. Readers in WA should check the current timeline, as the commencement date isn't yet locked in.

Once you're pursuing altruistic surrogacy: intended parents and the surrogate each get independent legal and counselling advice, and a written agreement is put in place before conception.

This catches many people off-guard, but legally, **the surrogate is recognised as the child's parent at birth**, regardless of genetic connection, until a court-issued parentage order transfers legal parentage afterward. This area of law is actively under national review by the Australian Law Reform Commission. Check current developments rather than relying only on this chapter, since it's one of the fastest-moving legal areas in this book.

If you're considering surrogacy overseas

Given commercial surrogacy is illegal everywhere in Australia, a lot of intended parents for whom altruistic surrogacy hasn't been possible to arrange here end up looking at international programs. The options, costs, and risks vary enormously by country and shift often.

Where Australians are currently going. The United States has the most established, well-regulated commercial surrogacy market in the world, with strong legal protections for intended parents in most states. However, it's also the most expensive option, with full programs commonly running close to AUD 150,000 or more.

Canada runs on an altruistic-only model similar to Australia's, but unlike Australia it has built significant infrastructure, such as agencies and matching services, around that model. This makes it easier to find a surrogate than in Australia, though it can still involve a long wait to be matched.

Colombia and Mexico have grown quickly as lower-cost destinations, particularly for same-sex couples, with total program costs commonly landing somewhere between AUD 80,000 and 150,000, though the legal landscape in both is still developing and can shift with little notice.

A caution on other destinations. Georgia, once popular, has faced repeated threats of restricting access to international patients, and "travelling surrogate" arrangements there have raised real ethical concerns.

Ukraine, a major destination before 2022, is now considered legally unpredictable and unsafe by surrogacy lawyers who previously recommended it.

A handful of lower-cost destinations exist elsewhere, but come with real risk: unclear legal processes, inconsistent medical standards, and difficulty securing your child's citizenship and safe exit from the country.

Citizenship isn't automatic. A child born overseas via surrogacy doesn't automatically become an Australian citizen. You'll need to apply for citizenship by descent and a passport, supported by legal documentation proving parentage. This process varies by destination country and can take weeks to arrange before you're able to bring your child home.

Engage a lawyer who specialises specifically in international surrogacy and Australian citizenship law before signing anything. Costs, legal frameworks, and even which countries are currently viable change often enough that anything written here should be treated as a starting point for that conversation, not the final word. Australia's own surrogacy laws are also under formal government review as this book is written, which may eventually change what's possible domestically.

Chapter Nineteen

Fertility Preservation

This chapter covers the two situations where fertility preservation most commonly occurs: freezing eggs, sperm, or embryos before a medical treatment that might affect your fertility, and freezing eggs electively, sometimes called "social" egg freezing, as a deliberate choice to preserve options for later.

They're clinically similar processes with very different cost structures, Medicare treatment, and emotional context, so it helps to understand them separately.

Medical fertility preservation

This applies when a treatment or condition threatens your future fertility, and you're freezing eggs, sperm, or embryos in response to that specific threat: most commonly before chemotherapy or radiation for a cancer diagnosis, but also relevant for some other medical treatments, and for trans and gender-diverse people preparing for gender-affirming hormone therapy or surgery.

This is the category where Medicare rebates actually apply, covering a meaningful portion of the cycle fee, medication, and hospital and anaesthetic costs. Several major clinics also offer priority access and reduced fees specifically for oncology patients. Bulk-billed initial consultations and discounted or waived storage fees are both fairly common, given the time pressure this group is usually under. If your situation involves a medical diagnosis affecting fertility, raise fertility preservation with your treating specialist (oncologist or otherwise) as early as possible, since chemotherapy and radiation timelines often don't allow much room to delay.

Elective egg freezing

This is a deliberate choice to freeze eggs while you're younger, without an immediate medical reason, to preserve the option of using your own eggs later: whether because you haven't met a partner, aren't ready yet, or simply want to reduce age-related pressure on a future decision.

Elective freezing attracts **no Medicare rebate** at all. Medications are still PBS-subsidised regardless of the reason for the cycle, but everything else is full out-of-pocket cost.

Typical cost: a single elective egg freezing cycle across major Australian providers commonly runs somewhere in the **$4,500-5,400** range, before medication (typically an additional **$1,000-1,500** or so) and before ongoing storage fees, which generally run **$275-500 per six months to a year**, depending on the clinic. There's no legal limit on how long eggs can be stored in Australia, provided consent is kept current, so this is a real, long-term, ongoing cost to budget for.

The statistics on what freezing your eggs actually buys you

This is the part worth reading slowly, because "egg freezing" is sometimes marketed, informally, as a kind of fertility insurance policy, and the real picture is more specific and more age-dependent than that framing suggests.

Age at freezing is the single biggest factor. Rough, commonly cited figures: eggs frozen before 35 carry approximately a 30-40% chance of a resulting baby per thaw cycle; 35-37 drops to approximately 20-30%; 38-40 to approximately 10-20%; over 40, under 10%. In summary, the earlier the eggs are frozen, the better the odds when they're eventually used.

The number of eggs matters as much as age. A commonly cited target for a reasonable chance of a future live birth is somewhere around 15-20 frozen eggs, which very often means more than one collection cycle, particularly for women in their late 30s who tend to produce fewer eggs per cycle than younger women. It's worth going into this with that expectation from the outset, rather than assuming a single cycle will necessarily be enough. This materially affects the total realistic cost, not just the headline single-cycle price above.

The actual live-birth rate from a frozen ("vitrified") egg, once thawed and fertilised, is broadly similar to the rate from a fresh egg used in a standard IVF cycle. The freezing and storage process itself isn't the weak link. Rather, it's the egg's age at the point of freezing that mostly determines the outcome.

Overall combined figures from Australian and New Zealand fertility preservation data put the total chance of eventually having a baby via this pathway at somewhere in the order of 25-40%, depending heavily on age at freezing and number of eggs collected. That is, it's a meaningful chance, but it's not a guarantee. Framing elective egg freezing as a definite safety net rather than a way of improving your odds can set up an unfair expectation later.

Eggs versus embryos

If you're in a stable relationship and comfortable using a partner's sperm now, some people choose to freeze **embryos** (fertilised eggs) rather than unfertilised eggs, since embryo survival and thaw rates are generally considered to be even better established than unfertilised egg vitrification.

The trade-off is that embryos are, by definition, linked to that specific partner, meaning you'll need their consent to use the embryos. Circumstances and relationships can change between freezing and eventual use, and eggs frozen unfertilised keep that specific decision open for later.

The decision itself

Whether elective freezing is worth it for you is a deeply personal calculation involving your age, your finances, your relationship status, and how much the "keeping options open" value matters to you specifically, weighed honestly against the real cost and the real, age-dependent odds above. A proper conversation with a fertility specialist, including your own AMH and antral follicle count results, will give you a far more personalised picture than the population-level ranges in this chapter.

Part Four

The Human Side

Chapter Twenty

Grief and Staying Connected as Partners

For me, infertility turned everything I thought I knew about what I wanted on its head. I was this high achieving, career focused woman who was so used to getting anything I wanted if I worked hard enough for it. Turns out, starting a family isn't so linear.

I was the only person in my peer group struggling to conceive. Pregnancy announcements kept arriving, one after another, from friends who I didn't even know were trying. I stopped turning up to baby showers, always with some lame excuse that I felt sounded reasonable enough at the time. I didn't buy presents for my friends' kids at Christmas. I just couldn't deal with it. Looking back now, I feel some shame about that version of myself. But at the time, the weight of being unable to conceive was so heavy that avoiding anything that touched it felt like the only way to keep functioning.

In some strange way, IVF was a reprieve from the uncertainty, because it gave me something to do: tests to investigate, a transfer to work toward, a sense that I could take control of a situation that had felt entirely outside my hands. But it came with its own challenges: the needles, the constant monitoring and the mounting bills.

This chapter is about acknowledging that grief, the isolation and the way it reshapes your relationships and your sense of yourself, because it is such a huge part of this journey.

A pain akin to cancer

Australian data, drawn from the Australian Longitudinal Study on Women's Health, found that half of women reporting either primary or secondary infertility also reported psychological distress, with the odds of that distress meaningfully higher than for women with no fertility difficulties.

Furthermore, levels of distress remained elevated even among women whose infertility had since resolved, meaning the impact doesn't simply switch off once treatment ends or a pregnancy happens. Separate reviews of the broader research literature report depression affecting somewhere between approximately 30 and 60 percent of women experiencing infertility, and anxiety somewhere between approximately 25 and 75 percent.

Perhaps the single most-cited finding in this field, repeated across multiple independent studies, is this: **the psychological distress associated with infertility has been found to be comparable to that experienced by people facing serious, life-threatening illnesses, cancer included.** It's a startling thing to read, and it's also, I think, exactly the kind of validation a lot of people going through this never get from the people around them.

Why it so often goes unrecognised

Infertility-related grief is frequently what's described as **disenfranchised grief**: a loss not widely acknowledged or socially sanctioned as grief at all. There's no funeral, no accepted ritual, often no shared language for what's been lost, and the loss itself (a future that hasn't happened, a child who was never conceived, or one conceived and then lost early) doesn't fit the picture of grief most people recognise and know how to support.

This helps explain a pattern a lot of people describe: friends and family who would show up without hesitation for almost any other kind of loss instead go quiet, say the wrong thing, or unintentionally minimise what's happening, not out of unkindness, but because the loss doesn't register to them as one.

If you have secondary infertility i.e. you are unable to conceive or carry a pregnancy to term after a previous successful pregnancy, you may have even less support that someone experiencing primary infertility. Friends, family, and sometimes even healthcare providers can unintentionally minimise what you're going through.

"At least you already have one."

"Just be grateful for what you've got."

"Some people can't have any."

These comments, almost always meant kindly, can still land as dismissive of a real and specific grief.

There's a particular kind of isolation that comes with this too: the friends who were your support network through your first pregnancy or fertility journey are sometimes the same people now unintentionally triggering pain, whether it's another pregnancy announcement, a sibling playdate, a well-meaning "when's baby number two coming?" It's common to feel a pull away from previously close relationships during this time, not because anything's wrong with them, but because proximity to what you're grieving is hard to sit inside.

How grief develops over time

Research into how infertility-related grief actually moves through a person describes it as cyclical rather than linear.

The grief is amplified at each negative test, each cycle, each pregnancy announcement from someone else, rather than following the more familiar stages-of-grief arc that gradually resolves toward acceptance. That's why it may feel like you're grieving the same loss repeatedly rather than moving steadily through it and out the other side.

The toll on relationships

Studies comparing infertile couples with fertile control groups have found lower marital adjustment scores among women specifically, alongside broader findings that both partners' individual stress levels affect not just their own relationship satisfaction, but their partner's.

A consistent pattern across multiple studies is that women and men often experience and express this differently. Women more frequently report the infertility itself as a source of distress to their sense of identity and wellbeing; men more frequently report a decline in sexual satisfaction specifically, sometimes attributed to the psychological pressure of performing on a schedule dictated by ovulation timing or clinic appointments rather than intimacy. Sex becoming task-based, tied to fertile windows and procedure dates rather than connection, is one of the most commonly reported strains on a relationship during this process, for both partners, in different ways.

None of this means infertility ruins relationships as a rule. Plenty of couples describe the experience as ultimately strengthening their relationship, not just straining it, and some research has found real relationship benefit reported specifically by women navigating this.

What the research more consistently points to is that how a couple communicates through it matters more than the infertility itself in determining relationship satisfaction. Stronger predictors of relationship wellbeing include openness between partners, and each partner's felt sense of the other's support.

What seems to help

The same body of research that documents how hard this is also points to what tends to ease it. Structured psychological support, such as cognitive behavioural therapy and couples counselling, has real, demonstrated efficacy in reducing distress during treatment, and some research even suggests a possible link between reduced distress and improved treatment outcomes.

Despite this, uptake of psychological support remains low. Fewer than one in ten people experiencing significant infertility-related distress actually access psychiatric or psychological support, perhaps indicating the undeserved shame that comes with infertility.

Staying connected as partners

Below are some practical tips if you are navigating IVF with your partner.

Different coping styles are normal. One of the most common sources of friction isn't disagreement about the goal; it's discovering you and your partner process this differently, and mistaking that for distance or a lack of care. One partner wants to talk through every detail immediately; the other needs quiet processing time first. One researches obsessively; the other prefers not to know more than necessary. Neither style is wrong, and acknowledging the difference explicitly avoids each partner privately reading the other's style as a lack of investment.

Contain the conversation rather than letting it take over. Couples who let fertility talk happen at any moment tend to find it consumes the relationship. A regular, dedicated check-in for treatment updates and feelings, rather than constantly talking about it, may help. So does splitting logistics (one partner handles clinic communication, the other handles billing) so the mental load doesn't default to one person.

On sex, specifically. When intercourse is timed to ovulation, or intimacy gets wrapped up in monitoring appointments and procedure dates, sex very commonly starts feeling like a scheduled task rather than connection. It may help to deliberately protect some intimacy that has nothing to do with conception, non-sexual touch, or simply saying out loud that sex has started to feel like a chore, so it doesn't quietly erode unacknowledged.

Stay a team, even when the physical burden isn't shared equally. One partner is often carrying more of it (the injections, the appointments, the procedures), and it's easy for that imbalance to tip into the other partner feeling sidelined, or the partner doing the physical work feeling like it's entirely theirs to carry alone. Attend appointments together where you can, stay properly informed rather than just being present, and check in on how the non-carrying partner is doing too. And watch for blame creeping in either direction, toward whichever partner's diagnosis is the identified factor, or toward yourself if it's yours. This is happening to both of you, not something one of you is doing to the other.

Set limits together. Partners sometimes discover, well into treatment, that they'd quietly been holding different limits about the number of cycles to try the whole time, and it surfaces at exactly the wrong moment, mid-crisis, rather than a calmer one where it could've been talked through properly. Revisit it together periodically, not just once at the start.

Bring in outside support before it feels like an emergency. If communication feels like it's breaking down, whether it keeps going in circles, or either of you is feeling like you're consistently unheard, a therapist experienced specifically in fertility is worth seeking out directly. Every Australian fertility clinic has counselling available as standard care, and using it isn't a sign the relationship is failing. This is, after all, one of the hardest things you'll experience as a couple.

Chapter Twenty-One

Telling the People Around You and the Impact of Faith

Australian research commissioned by Monash IVF found that fewer than one in ten women would feel comfortable telling their boss or colleagues they were struggling to conceive.

Work is often the hardest call, because career perception, scheduling, and privacy all collide at once. It's against the law in Australia for an employer to treat you less favourably because of an intention to become pregnant, which extends to fertility treatment. That protection doesn't remove the understandable, informal worry a lot of people still carry.

If you choose not to disclose, have a practical plan ready rather than improvising to reduce any anxiety about it. Telling a manager or HR only that you're dealing with a private medical matter, without specifics, is a commonly used approach. You're not obliged to say more, and most managers won't push once told something is private. Ask your clinic if they can provide medical certificates for appointments if your workplace wants documentation.

If you do choose to disclose, even just to one trusted colleague, it can make scheduling much easier without a broader announcement. Patient surveys often find people who did disclose more widely describe unexpected support.

Check whether your workplace expects standard sick or personal leave to cover appointments, or has a dedicated fertility leave policy. This varies hugely by employer and increasingly by state. New South Wales became the first state to introduce paid fertility treatment leave for public servants (five days for teachers, nurses, and other government employees); other states and employers vary, so check your own workplace directly.

Family involves a different set of trade-offs. Ask yourself honestly: will telling this person actually give you support, or add a layer of anxious check-ins to manage on top of everything else? Can they hold difficult news without needing you to manage their reaction to it too? There's no rule that immediate family has to know before extended family, or that everyone needs the same level of detail. For example, depending on your relationship, you could tell your parents everything and your in-laws simply that you're "working on starting a family". If you do tell family, be specific about what kind of support you want, since people generally want to help but don't always know how without being told.

Friends sit in an odd middle ground. They're your peers, so they're the most likely to know what you're going through, and you'd more naturally want to confide in them. However, their own situation (already pregnant, struggling themselves, not wanting kids) can complicate things in ways work and family don't, precisely because they are typically at the same stage of life as you. It's hard not to compare yourself against them. It's common to feel a pull away from certain friendships during this period, especially around friends who are pregnant or parenting already. This doesn't have to be permanent or dramatic. Simply telling a friend you need a bit of space around baby topics for a while is often easier than quietly withdrawing without explanation.

There's no single right approach across any of these three groups. Revisiting the decision as you go, for example telling more people later, or fewer than planned, is a completely reasonable response to a process that keeps changing.

If faith is part of this conversation for you

For a lot of people, deciding to pursue IVF isn't purely a medical or financial decision. It sits alongside religious or spiritual beliefs, and navigating that honestly, with yourself and with family who share your faith, is its own real part of this journey.

Views amongst religions differ. The Catholic Church opposes IVF, primarily because it separates conception from the marital act and because standard treatment can involve embryos that aren't ultimately transferred. Catholic couples who pursue IVF anyway often describe real tension in reconciling their desire to start a family with their faith leaders' rejection of the technology that makes that possible for them.

Other Christian denominations vary widely, with many broadly supportive provided the treatment uses the couple's own genetic material and avoids embryo destruction.

Judaism is generally supportive of IVF, including by many Orthodox authorities, often framed around the commandment to have children, though donor conception may raise further questions.

Islam broadly permits IVF between married spouses, but most schools of thought prohibit third-party donor sperm, eggs, or surrogacy, since it's seen as introducing a genetic line outside the marriage.

Two issues come up across nearly every religion: the moral status of the embryo, and what happens to embryos not used. If your treatment produces more embryos than you ultimately need, the choice to keep them frozen indefinitely, donate them to another family or to research, or allow them to be discarded is one some faiths treat as morally significant. Similarly, if a cycle results in a multiple pregnancy and a doctor raises selective reduction as an option, this is an area where religious and personal views can diverge sharply, and it's far better to have thought this through, ideally with input from a faith leader if that matters to you, before you're facing the decision under pressure.

If your faith is a significant part of your life, it's worth having an honest conversation with a religious leader, ideally one with some familiarity with fertility ethics specifically, before treatment begins rather than partway through. Plenty of couples find a path that respects their beliefs without requiring them to give up on treatment altogether.

Chapter Twenty-Two

Support Networks

Every Australian fertility clinic has access to fertility counselling built into standard care, so simply call your clinic to arrange an appointment. Counsellors working in this specific space are typically members of **ANZICA** (the Australian and New Zealand Infertility Counsellors Association), clinical psychologists, psychologists, and social workers with specific training and experience in the emotional dimensions of fertility treatment.

The only situations where counselling is mandatory is if you are pursuing donor conception treatment, or if you are undergoing IVF in Victoria.

Medicare's Better Access initiative

If you have a diagnosed mental health condition (clinically significant anxiety or depression, for instance), Medicare's Better Access initiative provides a rebate for up to 10 individual and 10 group allied mental health sessions per calendar year, accessed through a GP mental health treatment plan.

Peer support

There's a particular kind of understanding that comes only from someone who's actually been through this. Your existing support network may not fully understand what you are going through, however well-intentioned they are.

Australian organisations specifically in this space include:

- **ACCESS Australia**: a long-running national organisation providing information, resources, and peer connection specifically for people experiencing infertility.

- **VARTA's support directory**: VARTA maintains a curated list of support services, including Donor Conceived Australia (DCA) for donor-conceived people specifically, and links to broader mental health services.
- **Pink Elephants Support Network**: specifically for early pregnancy loss, relevant if your fertility journey has included miscarriage.
- **Solo Mums by Choice Australia** and **Rainbow Families**, covered in earlier chapters respectively, for support specific to those paths.

Clinic-run communities are another option. Several major fertility clinics run closed, moderated Facebook groups exclusively for their own patients, offering a space to share experiences with people on a closely similar journey, sometimes even at the same clinic, without the noise of a fully open public forum.

Online communities

Broader online spaces such as Facebook groups, forums and Reddit communities can be a real source of comfort, particularly in the early hours of the morning when nobody else is awake to talk to.

Some people find them consistently helpful throughout treatment whilst others may find that at certain points, such as in the middle of a two-week-wait, or after a loss, the constant stream of others' updates becomes more agitating than soothing.

It should be noted that individual experiences shared in these spaces, however heartfelt, aren't clinical advice, and it's worth being wary of specific medical claims, protocol suggestions, or supplement recommendations that circulate in these spaces without an evidence base behind them.

If you're in crisis

If you require immediate support. **Lifeline** (13 11 14) offers 24/7 crisis support, **Beyond Blue** (1300 22 4636) provides mental health support and information, and if you or someone else is in danger, call **000**.

Chapter Twenty-Three

When to Consider Stopping, Pausing, or Exploring Alternatives

For one person, a single cycle (decided in advance, win or lose) is enough, and that boundary being clear before starting is itself part of what makes it bearable. For another, it's eight cycles, or more, and stopping before exhausting every reasonable option would feel like the wrong ending to their own story. Neither is more correct than the other. What matters is that the decision is actually yours, made with clear information, rather than one that happens to you by default because nobody thought it through.

Things to consider

Infertility can make people vulnerable to continuing treatment well past the point where it's realistically likely to succeed, driven by hope, fear of regret, hearing stories of against-the-odds success, or simply not having a clear moment to stop and reassess. It's a well-documented pattern, and researchers have specifically flagged the risk of overtreatment as something the field itself needs to guard against.

This is exactly why your specialist's honest, personalised assessment of your actual chances matters so much.

A few things worth noticing in yourself:

- **The financial picture has meaningfully changed**: not just "this is expensive," which was true from the start, but a real shift in what continuing would cost you elsewhere in your life.

- **The physical and emotional toll has stopped feeling survivable**, distinct from simply being hard. This is about whether it's become more than that for you specifically.
- **Your specialist's honest assessment of your chances has shifted meaningfully**, and continuing no longer gives you the same hope as when you started.
- **You notice you're continuing primarily out of fear of regret or momentum, rather than genuine belief this specific next step will help**. This is one of the most commonly reported reasons people keep going past what they'd otherwise choose.

None of these, alone, means it's time to stop. Together, or persistently, they're worth a real conversation with your specialist, your partner if you have one, and possibly a fertility counsellor.

A pause to recover financially, physically, or emotionally, is a completely legitimate choice, and it doesn't require justifying to anyone, including your clinic. Some people pause and return; some people pause and, in that space, find the answer to whether they want to return at all.

If you decide to stop

Fertility counsellors who work specifically in this space have pushed back on the idea that stopping treatment produces closure in the way that word usually implies, that is, a clean resolution, a door shutting neatly. For a process this prolonged and this emotionally layered, resolution in that tidy sense often isn't realistic, and expecting it can leave people feeling like they're grieving wrong when the feelings don't wrap up the way "closure" suggests they should.

What tends to help more isn't chasing closure but finding your own way to mark the decision. Some people describe intentional rituals: one couple, after deciding to stop, held a gathering that served as both a farewell to the process and a recognition of everything they'd been through to get there, taking back some agency over an ending that otherwise felt like it had been decided for them by circumstance rather than choice.

The alternatives that exist

If treatment ends without the outcome you were hoping for, several paths remain. However I won't pretend that these options "resolve" the grief of what didn't happen the way you'd originally hoped.

A child-free life can take different forms, whether it's actively deciding not to pursue further avenues, or a "not trying, not preventing" middle ground that some people find offers space and closure of its own. There's no obligation to explain or justify this choice to anyone.

Adoption is often assumed to be the natural next step after fertility treatment doesn't work. However according to the Australian Institute of Health and Welfare, adoptions in Australia have fallen 98 percent since their 1971-72 peak of 9,798 a year: down to 207 in 2023-24, and 155 in 2024-25, across the entire country. Of those, the clear majority are known child adoptions (a step-parent or existing carer, such as a foster parent, formalising a relationship with a child they already care for), not the kind of adoption most people picture when they imagine building a family this way. Local adoptions, where a child unrelated and previously unknown to the adoptive parents is placed with them, numbered in the dozens nationally, not hundreds.

Intercountry adoption has declined even further (down 92 percent from its 2004-05 peak of 434 to just 34 in 2023-24), and where it remains available, the median wait from application to placement is around three and a half to four years, with its own substantial cost (commonly quoted around $10,000 or more, on top of local adoption fees).

I want to be direct about what this means: adoption in Australia, for someone without an existing relationship to a specific child, is realistically not a readily available path, however much it's culturally assumed to be one. Going in with the expectation that adoption functions as a reliable "next step" after fertility treatment risks a further, compounding disappointment.

Donor conception or surrogacy, remain available options if your specific situation makes them relevant and appealing.

Fostering, though outside the scope of this book, is another path some people explore.

Part Five

After

Chapter Twenty-Four

If It Works: Pregnancy After IVF

I want to open this chapter by stating something that surprises a lot of people: a positive result doesn't switch off the fear that someone who has experienced infertility carries. For many people, it simply changes shape. This chapter is about the practical realities of pregnancy after IVF, and about how that fear shifts onto the pregnancy itself.

IVF and pregnancy risk

Most IVF pregnancies proceed and result in a healthy birth. That being said, this book has been consistent throughout about not softening real information, and the honest picture includes some meaningfully elevated risks that are worth knowing about, not to frighten you, but so nothing catches you or your care team off guard.

Systematic review evidence shows IVF pregnancies carry a somewhat higher rate of certain complications compared with pregnancies conceived without medical intervention: this includes an increased risk of stillbirth, and meta-analyses have found approximately 70% higher relative risk of pre-eclampsia and 25-50% higher relative risk of gestational diabetes. These are relative increases on figures that remain low in absolute terms, and they partly reflect the underlying factors that led to needing IVF in the first place (age, in particular) rather than something inherent to the IVF process itself. Nevertheless, additional monitoring is recommended for IVF pregnancies.

Miscarriage risk is highest in the earliest weeks and drops meaningfully once a pregnancy passes the 12-week mark. After this point, ongoing miscarriage risk in IVF pregnancies is typically around 2%, though your own risk depends on your specific history, age, and whether a genetically tested (PGT-A) embryo was used, which tends to further reduce this figure. If you have a history of miscarriage or recurrent loss, most clinics offer more frequent monitoring and specific miscarriage-care programs in a subsequent pregnancy.

Multiples carry meaningfully higher risk again. Twin pregnancies, IVF or otherwise, come with approximately four times the risk of maternal illness and perinatal complications compared with a singleton, and a considerably higher rate of preterm birth. This is one of several reasons single embryo transfer has become the standard recommended approach in Australia rather than transferring multiple embryos to improve odds, as was done historically.

The dating quirk

Standard pregnancy dating counts from the first day of your last period, but that reference point doesn't apply cleanly to an IVF pregnancy, where the actual date of fertilisation and transfer is known precisely. Make sure your embryo transfer date (and whether it was a day-3 or day-5 transfer) is clearly recorded and passed on to whichever care provider takes over from your fertility clinic: it directly affects your due date calculation and the timing of early scans.

The transition out of fertility care

During treatment, you've likely had frequent scans, regular bloodwork, and a clinical team who knew your specific case in detail, reachable directly with questions. Standard antenatal care, once you transition to a GP-shared care arrangement or an obstetrician, typically involves considerably less frequent contact: often a first obstetric appointment around 8-10 weeks, then approximately monthly visits through much of the pregnancy, without the reassurance scans you may have grown used to.

For a lot of people who've been through fertility treatment, this drop in monitoring intensity is one of the more anxiety-provoking parts of the whole process, because the rhythm of reassurance you'd adapted to simply isn't part of standard care.

A few practical things that help with this transition: ask your fertility clinic directly what they typically pass on to your ongoing care provider, rather than assuming it happens automatically. If your anxiety about the reduced monitoring feels like more than manageable worry, raise it directly with your GP or obstetrician as some will accommodate an additional early reassurance scan.

The anxiety that doesn't just disappear

This deserves to be said, because it often isn't: pregnancy after infertility and loss is not the same emotional experience as pregnancy without that history. Having been through failed cycles, or a chemical pregnancy, or pregnancy loss, tends to make the anxiety of early pregnancy sit differently, often more intensely, and for longer than the "first trimester and then it eases" pattern some pregnant people describe. If you find yourself unable to relax even with reassuring results, or bracing constantly against the possibility of loss well past the point your care team says risk has dropped, that's an extremely common response.

If this anxiety feels like it's taking over, raise it directly with your GP, obstetrician, or mental health service.

PANDA (Perinatal Anxiety & Depression Australia) operates Australia's only National Perinatal Mental Health Helpline (1300 726 306) that specifically supports perinatal mental health.

The end of fertility treatment doesn't mean the end of needing, or deserving, support for the emotional weight of what got you here.

Chapter Twenty-Five

If It Doesn't Work: Rebuilding and Redefining What Comes Next

This chapter is about what comes after the decision has been made to stop, pause, or change course - not the moment of it, but the months and years that follow, when treatment is no longer the organising fact of your life and something else has to take its place.

What the research shows

A qualitative study following women an average of nearly four years after unsuccessful treatment described their experience using two words that don't usually sit together: loss and opportunity. Both dimensions were present, at once, in the same accounts: not loss followed eventually by opportunity, but both, often at once, shaping an altered but not diminished sense of self.

More encouraging still, a 10-year follow-up study comparing childless couples with couples who went on to have children after treatment found that there was no statistically significant difference in overall life satisfaction, relationship satisfaction, friendship satisfaction, or sexual satisfaction between the two groups a decade on. Childless women in that study actually reported *higher* occupational satisfaction than mothers did. This doesn't erase the real grief, but it does show that a full, satisfying life on the other side of unsuccessful treatment isn't just possible in the abstract; it's what actually tends to happen, over time, for most people.

Why this doesn't feel true in the early aftermath

None of this means the early period after stopping feels easy. The research describes an *adjustment process*, not an instant shift. Clinical frameworks used by reproductive mental health professionals describe stages that echo general grief work: denial, anger, a bargaining pull back toward "just one more try," a period of real sadness and withdrawal, and eventually something closer to integration, where the experience becomes part of your story without needing to be erased or constantly relived. These stages aren't linear, and moving between them, sometimes backward, isn't a sign you're doing this wrong. "Closure" in the tidy sense often isn't realistic for a loss this prolonged, and that holds just as true in the months and years afterward as it did in the moment of deciding to stop.

Research specifically on the psychological process of this adjustment has found something practically useful: letting go of the specific parenting goals treatment was built around, and finding new meaning that isn't contingent on reaching them, is associated with better emotional adjustment over time than continuing to hold those exact goals in an unresolved, unattainable way. This isn't the same as suppressing grief or pretending the original hope didn't matter; it's closer to what the earlier qualitative research called integration: the loss becomes part of a coherent life story rather than a permanent unresolved fracture running underneath everything else.

After an extended period of treatment, some people describe a kind of disconnection from their own body: a coping mechanism that made sense during invasive procedures and repeated disappointment, but which can persist afterward as numbness or detachment long after appointments have ended. Reconnecting with your body and your broader identity, beyond whatever it did or didn't achieve in treatment, is often described as a meaningful part of this adjustment period, not something that simply resolves on its own with time alone.

Practical support for this specific phase

A few things worth specifically seeking out for this phase:

- **A reproductive mental health professional**, distinct from general grief counselling, who understands the specific experience of infertility, pregnancy loss and treatment ending.
- **A peer community specifically for people beyond active treatment**, rather than the treatment-focused forums and groups covered earlier in this book. The concerns are different at this stage, and being surrounded by people still mid-cycle can make an already isolating adjustment feel harder rather than easier.
- **A plan for the practical loose ends**, embryo storage decisions, cancelling autopay on medication or storage fees, closing out clinic paperwork, so the administrative tail of treatment doesn't keep resurfacing the decision every time a bill or reminder arrives.
- **Space for your partner's version of this**, if you have one. Grief around stopping treatment doesn't always arrive on the same timeline for both people.
- **A GP follow-up**, particularly if the physical side of treatment, medication, procedures, the toll on your body, hasn't had a proper close-out conversation, or if you need additional psychological support.

Conclusion

There is no single ending this book is steering you toward.

There's just your situation, your body, your finances, your relationships, and the decisions that only you and the people closest to you can make.

What I can tell you, from the other side of my own journey, is that the process itself changes you regardless of how it ends. You'll likely know yourself and your limits better than you ever expected to. You'll probably have hard conversations, with partners, with family, with friends that you wouldn't have had otherwise. Some of that is incredibly difficult. But some of it is also, unexpectedly, a kind of clarity: about what you actually want and what a full life can look like even when it doesn't arrive by the route you first imagined.

Whatever your own story becomes - whether it's a child conceived on the first cycle, or the tenth; donor conception; a decision to stop; a life built without a child that turns out to be full in ways you can't yet picture from where you're standing now - I hope this book has given you a clearer understanding of the journey to meet whatever ending arrives.

Glossary of Key Terms

Add-ons

Optional (or sometimes clinically necessary) extras offered alongside a standard IVF cycle, such as ICSI and PGT-A usually priced separately from the core cycle fee.

Adenomyosis

A condition in which tissue similar to the uterine lining grows into the muscular wall of the uterus, which can affect fertility and implantation.

Agonist protocol ("long protocol")

A stimulation protocol in which a GnRH agonist (e.g. Lucrin, Synarel, Decapeptyl) is used first to temporarily switch off the natural hormone cycle - down-regulation - before stimulation begins. Takes longer and involves more medication than the antagonist protocol, but gives the clinic more complete control over timing; often chosen for endometriosis or a poor response to the antagonist protocol.

AMH (Anti-Müllerian Hormone) test

A blood test that estimates ovarian reserve.

Aneuploid

A PGT-A result showing an embryo has an abnormal number of chromosomes, meaning that it is unlikely to result in a live birth.

Antagonist protocol

The most common default stimulation protocol: FSH stimulation starts early in the cycle, and an antagonist medication (e.g. Cetrotide or Orgalutran) is added partway through to prevent early ovulation before retrieval. Shorter than the agonist protocol, with a lower risk of OHSS.

Antral follicle count

An ultrasound measure of the small follicles visible in the ovaries at the start of a cycle, used alongside AMH as a marker of ovarian reserve.

ART (Assisted Reproductive Technology)

The umbrella term for medical procedures used to achieve pregnancy, including IVF, ICSI, and related treatments.

Blastocyst

The stage an embryo reaches by day five or six of culture - a larger, more complex structure of hundreds of cells, and the point at which embryos are typically transferred or frozen.

Conventional insemination

The standard IVF fertilisation method in which eggs and prepared sperm are placed together in a dish and allowed to fertilise on their own, as distinct from ICSI.

Donor conception

Using donor eggs, sperm, or embryos to conceive.

Down-regulation

The temporary suppression of the natural hormone cycle using a GnRH agonist, used at the start of an agonist ("long") protocol before ovarian stimulation begins.

Egg (oocyte) retrieval / egg pick-up (EPU)

The day-surgery procedure, done under sedation or light anaesthetic, in which a fine needle is passed through the vaginal wall to draw eggs from the ovarian follicles.

Embryo transfer

The procedure in which a single embryo is placed into the uterus via a thin catheter, either fresh (around day five after retrieval) or frozen (in a later FET cycle).

EMSN (Extended Medicare Safety Net)

A Medicare safety net that tracks the full out-of-pocket gap between what a clinic charges and what Medicare pays; once a calendar-year threshold is reached, Medicare's rebate for further services increases.

Endometriosis

A condition in which tissue similar to the uterine lining grows outside the uterus, which can affect fertility and - where tubes are blocked - may make IUI unsuitable and IVF the more appropriate step. Surgical treatment sometimes resolves the issue enough that no further assisted treatment is needed; in other cases, it's a reason a specialist may recommend the agonist ("long") stimulation protocol.

ERA (Endometrial Receptivity Analysis)

A test sometimes used to assess whether the uterine lining is at its optimal window for embryo transfer, referenced among add-on options for people with previous unsuccessful transfers.

Euploid

A PGT-A result showing an embryo has the correct (normal) number of chromosomes - the result associated with the best chance of implanting and developing normally.

FET (Frozen Embryo Transfer)

A cycle in which a previously frozen embryo is thawed and transferred, prepared either naturally (tracking the body's own cycle) or with medication.

Fertilisation check

The lab assessment, approximately 16-18 hours after insemination or ICSI, that looks for two pronuclei (2PN) which is the sign that sperm and egg have combined.

Fibroids

Non-cancerous growths in or on the uterus, checked for during the initial pelvic ultrasound. Can be a contributing factor in both primary and secondary infertility, and are sometimes treated surgically before or alongside fertility treatment.

Freeze-all cycle

A cycle in which every viable embryo is frozen at the blastocyst stage rather than transferred fresh, with the transfer happening later in a separate FET cycle - often used to reduce OHSS risk or await PGT-A results.

Fresh transfer

An embryo transfer that happens around day five after egg retrieval, in the same stimulated cycle, rather than in a later frozen cycle.

FSH (Follicle-Stimulating Hormone)

A hormone measured by blood test, usually early in the cycle, as part of assessing ovulation function and ovarian reserve.

HSG (Hysterosalpingogram)

An X-ray or ultrasound-based procedure that checks whether the fallopian tubes are open and the uterine cavity is a normal shape.

ICSI (Intracytoplasmic Sperm Injection)

A fertilisation technique in which an embryologist injects a single sperm directly into each mature egg, typically used to address male-factor infertility.

IUI (Intrauterine Insemination)

A fertility treatment in which prepared sperm is placed directly into the uterus around ovulation, often used as a step before moving to IVF.

IVF (In-Vitro Fertilisation)

The core treatment covered by this book: eggs and sperm are combined outside the body, and a resulting embryo is transferred to the uterus.

LH (Luteinising Hormone)

A hormone measured alongside FSH in initial fertility bloodwork to assess ovulation function.

Luteal support

Progesterone supplementation (pessary, injection, or oral medication) given after embryo transfer to help sustain the uterine lining through early implantation.

Mini-IVF / natural cycle IVF

A stimulation approach using little or no stimulation medication, working with the single egg the body would produce naturally, or a very small, mildly stimulated number. Chosen far less often, for a specific medical reason or personal preference, with lower success rates per cycle than conventional stimulation.

Mosaic embryo

An embryo whose PGT-A result shows a mixture of chromosomally normal and abnormal cells, as distinct from a clearly euploid (normal) or aneuploid (abnormal) result.

OHSS (Ovarian Hyperstimulation Syndrome)

A condition in which the ovaries respond more strongly than intended to stimulation medication, causing swelling and, in more significant cases, fluid leakage into the abdomen.

OMSN (Original Medicare Safety Net)

The smaller of the two Medicare safety nets, tracking the gap between the standard 85% rebate and 100% of the schedule fee; once a calendar-year threshold is reached, the rebate rises to 100%.

PBS (Pharmaceutical Benefits Scheme)

The government scheme that subsidises the cost of prescription medications, including many IVF medications, once patients meet certain criteria.

PBS Safety Net

A threshold of PBS medication spending in a calendar year, after which the cost of further PBS medications drops significantly (or becomes free for concession card holders).

PCOS (Polycystic Ovary Syndrome)

A common hormonal condition that can affect ovulation and is associated with a higher risk of OHSS during stimulated IVF cycles.

PESA (Percutaneous Epididymal Sperm Aspiration)

A needle-based procedure used to retrieve sperm directly from the epididymis, typically used where sperm production is normal but a blockage prevents sperm from reaching the ejaculate.

PGT-A (Preimplantation Genetic Testing for Aneuploidy)

A test in which cells biopsied from a developing embryo (usually at blastocyst stage) are screened for the correct number of chromosomes before a transfer decision, typically priced per embryo and not Medicare-rebated.

PGT-M / PGT-SR

Related preimplantation genetic tests used to check embryos for a known single-gene condition (PGT-M) or a structural chromosome rearrangement (PGT-SR) running in a family, as distinct from general PGT-A screening.

PICSI (Physiological Intracytoplasmic Sperm Injection)

A sperm-selection technique used alongside ICSI, in which sperm are selected based on their ability to bind to a substance mimicking the egg's outer layer.

RTAC (Reproductive Technology Accreditation Committee)

The body, sitting under the Fertility Society of Australia and New Zealand, that accredits Australian fertility clinics.

Secondary infertility

The inability to conceive or carry a pregnancy to term after a previous successful pregnancy, affecting approximately one in ten couples trying for another child.

Stimulation (ovarian stimulation)

The phase of an IVF cycle, typically days one to twelve, in which injectable hormone medications are used to encourage the ovaries to develop multiple mature follicles.

Surrogacy

An arrangement in which another person carries and gives birth to a child on behalf of intended parent(s).

TESE (Testicular Sperm Extraction)

A surgical procedure used to retrieve sperm directly from the testicle, typically used where sperm is absent from the ejaculate.

Trigger shot (trigger injection)

An injection of hCG (sometimes combined with another medication) given once lead follicles reach maturity, completing final egg maturation and precisely timing ovulation ahead of egg retrieval.

Two-week wait

The approximately nine-to-fourteen-day period between embryo transfer and a blood (beta hCG) test that can reliably confirm whether implantation has occurred.

YourIVFSuccess / ANZARD

YourIVFSuccess is the Australian Government-funded national IVF success-rate estimator tool, operated by UNSW's National Perinatal Epidemiology and Statistics Unit (NPESU), drawing on data from the Australian and New Zealand Assisted Reproduction Database (ANZARD).

Index

Key Sources

I have listed below the key Australian sources I referred to, organised by chapter. If any of these topics are relevant for you, check them directly for anything current or specific to your situation, since costs, government rebates, and regulations shift over time.

I have not included links to information published in relation to IVF overseas, or on clinic websites, comparison sites, and professional and personal blogs.

Chapter One: Is It Time?

- Your Fertility - Trying-to-conceive guidance: https://www.yourfertility.org.au
- healthdirect - Partner page for Your Fertility: https://www.healthdirect.gov.au/partners/your-fertility
- Services Australia - Referrals for specialist treatment: https://www.servicesaustralia.gov.au/referrals-for-specialist-treatment

Chapter Three: Common Myths about IVF in Australia

- NCBI/PubMed - High and growing disapproval of sex-selection technology in Australia: https://www.ncbi.nlm.nih.gov/pmc/articles/PMC6125943/
- NCBI/PubMed - Regulation of assisted reproductive treatment (ART) in Australia & current ethical issues: https://pmc.ncbi.nlm.nih.gov/articles/PMC4345760/

Chapter Four: Choosing a Clinic

- YourIVFSuccess - The Australian Government-funded national IVF success rate and estimator tool: https://yourivfsuccess.com.au

- Australian and New Zealand Assisted Reproduction Database (ANZARD): https://www.unsw.edu.au/research/npesu/clinical-registries/anz-assisted-reproduction-database

Chapter Five: Understanding Your Diagnosis (Or the Absence of One)

- Victorian Department of Health - Public Fertility Care access criteria, including age cutoffs: https://www.health.vic.gov.au/public-health/public-fertility-care
- Royal Women's Hospital - Public Fertility Care eligibility, donor egg age requirements: https://www.thewomens.org.au/patients-visitors/clinics-and-services/fertility-genetics/public-fertility-services
- healthdirect - Infertility prevalence: https://www.healthdirect.gov.au/about-infertility
- FSANZ – Female infertility: https://www.fertilitysociety.com.au/resources/female-infertility/
- Healthy Male - Male infertility: https://healthymale.org.au/mens-health/infertility

Chapter Six: Medicare and the Real Cost of IVF in Australia

- Services Australia - MBS billing rules for Assisted Reproductive Technology services: https://www.servicesaustralia.gov.au/mbs-billing-for-assisted-reproductive-technology-services
- Services Australia - Medicare Safety Nets, registration, and thresholds: https://www.servicesaustralia.gov.au/medicare-safety-nets
- Services Australia - PBS Safety Net thresholds, effective 1 January 2026: https://www.servicesaustralia.gov.au/pbs-safety-net-thresholds
- NSW Health - NSW Affordable IVF Initiative: https://www.health.nsw.gov.au/kidsfamilies/MCFhealth/maternity/Pages/affordable-IVF.aspx

- VIC Department of Health - Public Fertility Care eligibility and service model: https://www.health.vic.gov.au/public-health/public-fertility-care

Chapter Eight: What Private Health Insurance Covers

- Private Health Insurance Ombudsman - Private Health Insurance factsheet on Assisted Reproductive Services: https://www.ombudsman.gov.au/publications-and-news-pages/publication-pages/brochures-and-factsheets/factsheets/private-health-insurance/assisted-reproductive-services
- PBS - PBS-subsidised IVF medicines: https://www.pbs.gov.au/browse/section100/ivf-program

Chapter Nine: Budgeting and Financing More Than One Cycle

- ATO - Early release of superannuation on compassionate grounds: https://www.ato.gov.au/individuals-and-families/super-for-individuals-and-families/super/withdrawing-and-using-your-super/early-access-to-super/access-on-compassionate-grounds/eligible-expenses-for-compassionate-release-of-super/medical-treatment#EvidenceforinvitrofertilisationIVF

Chapter Sixteen: When a Cycle Doesn't Work: What Happens Next

- Evidence-based IVF, University of Melbourne - Independent add-on evidence resource: https://www.unimelb.edu.au/ivf

Chapter Eighteen: Donor Conception and Surrogacy

- VARTA - Donor conception explained: https://www.varta.org.au/understanding-donor-conception/donor-conception-explained
- NSW Health - The Central Register: https://www.health.nsw.gov.au/art/Pages/the-central-register.aspx

Chapter Twenty-Two: Support Networks

- VARTA - Additional support directory: https://www.varta.org.au/resources/support

- Gidget Foundation - Conception and fertility difficulties: https://www.gidgetfoundation.org.au/becoming-a-parent/conception-and-fertility-difficulties

Chapter Twenty-Three: When to Consider Stopping, Pausing, or Exploring Alternatives

- VARTA - Deciding to stop IVF treatment, first-person account and personal story series: https://www.varta.org.au/resources/personal-stories/deciding-stop-ivf-treatment

- AIHW - Australian Institute of Health and Welfare - Australian Adoptions Data: https://www.aihw.gov.au/reports-data/health-welfare-services/adoptions/overview

Chapter Twenty-Four: If It Works: Pregnancy After IVF

- Safer Care Victoria - In vitro fertilization (IVF) and pregnancy risk: https://www.safercare.vic.gov.au/publications/in-vitro-fertilization-ivf-and-pregnancy-risk

About the author

L. C. Hughes is the pen name of an Australian lawyer who went through IVF after being diagnosed with unexplained infertility, and struggled to find honest, Australia-specific information along the way. *The IVF Roadmap* is the book she wished had existed back then.

She lives in Sydney with her husband and their two kids, and still can't quite believe that she gets to write that sentence.